Contents

A Concise Guide to Clinical Trials

Allan Hackshaw

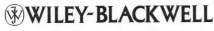
WILEY-BLACKWELL

A John Wiley & Sons, Ltd., Publication

BMJ | Books

Preface

Clinical trials have revolutionised the way disease is prevented, detected or treated, and early death avoided. They continue to be an expanding area of research. They are central to the work of pharmaceutical companies, which cannot make a claim about a new drug or medical device until there is sufficient evidence on its efficacy. Trials originating from the academic or public sector are more common because they also evaluate existing therapies in different ways, or interventions that do not involve a commercial product.

Many health professionals are expected to conduct their own trials, or to participate in trials by recruiting subjects. They should have a sufficient understanding of the scientific and administrative aspects, including an awareness of the regulations and guidelines associated with clinical trials, which are now more stringent in many countries, making it more difficult to set up and run trials.

This book provides a comprehensive overview of the design, analysis and conduct of trials. It is aimed at health professionals and other researchers, and can be used as an introduction to clinical trials, as a teaching aid, or as a reference guide. No prior knowledge of trial design or conduct is required because the important concepts are presented throughout the chapters. References to each chapter and a reading list are provided for those who wish to learn more. Further details of trial set up and conduct can also be found from country-specific regulatory agencies.

The contents have come about through over 18 years of teaching epidemiology and medical statistics to undergraduates, postgraduates and health professionals, and designing, setting up and analysing clinical studies for a variety of disorders. Sections of this book have been based on successful short courses. This has all helped greatly in determining what researchers need to know, and how to present certain ideas. The book should be an easy-to-read guide to the topic.

I am most grateful to the following people for their helpful comments and advice on the text: Dhiraj Abhyankar, Roisin Cinneide, Hannah Farrant, Christine Godfrey, Nicole Gower, Michael Hughes, Naseem Kabir, Iftekhar Khan, Alicja Rudnicka, and in particular Roger A'Hern. Very special thanks go to Jan Mackie, whose thorough editing was invaluable. And final thanks go to Harald Bauer.

Allan Hackshaw
Deputy Director of the Cancer Research UK & UCL Cancer Trials Centre

Foreword

No one would doubt the importance of clinical trials in the progress and practice of medicine today. They have developed enormously over the last 60 years, and have made significant contributions to our knowledge about the efficacy of new treatments, particularly in quantifying the magnitude of their effects. Crucial in this development was the acceptance, albeit with considerable initial opposition, to randomisation – essentially tossing a coin to determine treatment allocation. Over the past 60 years clinical trials have become highly sophisticated, in their design, conduct, statistical analysis and the processes required before new medicines can be legally sold. They have become expensive and requiring large teams of experts covering pharmacology, mathematics, computing, health economics and epidemiology to mention only a few. The systematic combination of the results from many trials to provide clearer results, in the form of meta-analyses, have themselves developed their own sophistication and importance.

In all this panoply of activity and complexity it is easy to lose sight of the elements that form the basis of good science and practice in the conduct of clinical trials. Allan Hackshaw, in this book, achieves this with great skill. He informs the general reader of the essential elements of clinical trials; how they should be designed, how to calculate the number of people needed for such trials, the different forms of trial design, and importantly the recognition that a randomised clinical trial is not always the right way to obtain an answer to a particular medical question.

As well as dealing with the scientific issues, this book is useful in describing the terminology and procedures used in connection with clinical trials, including explanations of phase I, II, III and IV trials. The book describes the regulations governing the conduct of clinical trials and those that relate to the approval and sale of new medicines – an area that has become extremely complicated, with few people having a grasp of the "whole" picture.

This book educates the general medical and scientific reader on clinical trials without requiring detailed knowledge in any particular area. It provides an up to date overview of clinical trials with commendable clarity.

Professor Sir Nicholas Wald
Director, Wolfson Institute of Environmental & Preventive Medicine
Barts and The London School of Medicine & Dentistry

CHAPTER 1

Fundamental concepts

This chapter provides a brief background to clinical trials, and why they are considered to be the 'gold standard' in health research. This is followed by a summary of the main types of trials, and four key design features. Further details on design and analysis are given in Chapters 3–7.

1.1 What is a clinical trial?

There are two distinct study designs used in health research: observational and experimental (Box 1.1). Observational studies do not intentionally involve intervening in the way individuals live their lives, or how they are treated. However, clinical trials are specifically designed to intervene, and then evaluate some health-related outcome, with one or more of the following objectives:

- to diagnose or detect disease
- to treat an existing disorder
- to prevent disease or early death
- to change behaviour, habits or other lifestyle factors.

Some trials evaluate new drugs or medical devices that will later require a **licence** (or **marketing authorisation**) for human use from a regulatory authority, if a benefit is shown. This allows the treatment to be marketed and routinely available to the public. Other trials are based on therapies that are already licensed, but will be used in different ways, such as a different disease group, or in combination with other treatments.

An **intervention** could be a single **treatment** or **therapy**, namely an administered substance that is injected, swallowed, inhaled or absorbed through the skin; an exposure such as radiotherapy; a surgical technique; or a medical/dental device. A combination of interventions can be referred to as a **regimen**, such as, chemotherapy plus surgery in treating cancer. Other interventions could be educational or behavioural programmes, or dietary changes. Any administered drug or micronutrient that is examined in a clinical trial with the specific purpose of treating, preventing or diagnosing disease is usually referred to as an **Investigational Medicinal Product (IMP)** or **Investigational**

A concise guide to clinical trials, First edition. By A. Hackshaw. Published 2009 by Blackwell Publishing, ISBN: 978-1-4051-6774-1.

Box 1.1 Study designs in health research

Observational

Cross-sectional: compare the proportion of people with the disorder among those who are or are not exposed, at one point in time.

Case-control: take people with and without the disorder now, and compare the proportions that were or were not exposed in the past.

Cohort: take people without the disorder now, and ascertain whether they happen to be exposed or not. Then follow them up, and compare the proportions that develop the disorder in the future, among those who were or were not exposed.

Semi-experimental

Trials with historical controls: give the exposure to people now, and compare the proportion who develop the disorder with the proportion who were not exposed in the past.

Experimental

Randomised controlled trial: randomly allocate people to have the exposure or control now. Then follow them up, and compare the proportions that develop the disorder in the future between the two groups.

An 'exposure' could be a new treatment, and those 'not exposed' or in a control group could have been given standard therapy.

New Drug (IND).[#] An IMP could be a newly developed drug, or one that already is licensed for human use. Most clinical trial regulations that are part of law in several countries cover studies using an IMP, and sometimes medical devices.

Throughout this book, 'intervention', 'treatment' and 'therapy' are used interchangeably. People who take part in a trial are referred to as 'subjects' or 'participants' (if they are healthy individuals), or 'patients' (if they are already ill). They are allocated to trial or intervention arms or groups.

Well-designed clinical trials with a proper statistical analysis provide robust and objective evidence. One of the most important uses of evidence-based medicine is to determine whether a new intervention is more effective than another, or that it has a similar effect, but is safer, cheaper or more convenient to administer. It is therefore essential to have good evidence to decide whether it is appropriate to change practice.

[#] IMP in the European Union, and IND in the United States and Japan.

World Health Organization definition of a clinical trial[1,2]

Any research study that prospectively assigns human participants or groups of humans to one or more health-related interventions to evaluate the effects on health outcomes.

Health outcomes include any biomedical or health-related measures obtained in patients or participants, including pharmacokinetic measures and adverse events.

1.2 Early trials

James Lind, a Scottish naval physician, is regarded as conducting the first clinical trial.[3] During a sea voyage in 1747, he chose 12 sailors with similarly severe cases of scurvy, and examined six treatments, each given to two sailors: cider, diluted sulphuric acid, vinegar, seawater, a mixture of several foods including nutmeg and garlic, and oranges and lemons. They were made to live in the same part of the ship and with the same basic diet. Lind felt it was important to standardise their living conditions to ensure that any change in their disease is unlikely to be due to other factors. After about a week, both sailors given fruit had almost completely recovered, compared to little or no improvement in the other sailors. This dramatic effect led Lind to conclude that eating fruit was essential to curing scurvy, without knowing that it was specifically due to vitamin C. The results of his trial were supported by observations made by other seamen and physicians.

Lind had little doubt about the value of fruit. Two important features of his trial were: a **comparison** between two or more interventions, and an attempt to ensure that the subjects had **similar characteristics**. That the requirement for these two features has not changed is an indication of how important they are to conducting good trials that aim to provide reliable answers.

One key element missing from Lind's trial was the process of **randomisation**, whereby the decision on which intervention a subject receives cannot be influenced by the researcher or subject. An early attempt to do this appeared in a trial on diphtheria in 1898, which used day of admission to allocate patients to the treatments.[4] Those admitted on one day received the standard therapy, and those admitted on the subsequent day received the standard therapy plus a serum treatment. However, some physicians could have admitted patients with mild disease on the day when the serum treatment would be given, and this could bias the results in favour of this treatment. The Medical Research Council trial of streptomycin and tuberculosis in 1948 is regarded as the first to use random numbers.[5] Allocating subjects using a random number list meant that it was not possible to predict what treatment would be given to each patient, thus minimising the possibility of bias in the allocation.

1.3 Why are research studies, such as clinical trials, needed?

Smoking is a cause of lung cancer, and statin therapy is effective in treating coronary heart disease. However, why do some people who have smoked 40 cigarettes a day for life not develop lung cancer, while others who have never smoked a single cigarette do? Why do some patients who have had a heart attack and been given statin therapy have a second attack, while others do not. The answer is that people *vary*. They have different body characteristics (for example, weight, height, blood pressure and blood measurements), different genetic make-up and different lifestyles (for example, diet, exercise, and smoking and alcohol consumption habits). This is all referred to as **variability** or **natural variation.** People react to the same exposure or treatment in different ways; what may affect one person may not affect another. When a new intervention is evaluated, it is essential to consider if the observed responses are consistent with this natural variation, or whether there really is a treatment effect. Variability needs to be allowed for in order to judge how much of the difference seen at the end of a trial is due to natural variation (i.e. chance), and how much is due to the action of the new intervention. The more variability there is, the harder it is to see if a new treatment is effective. Detecting and measuring the effect of a new intervention in the setting of natural variation is the principal concern of medical statistics, used to design and analyse research studies.

Before describing the main design features of clinical trials, it is worth considering other types of studies that can assess the effectiveness of an intervention, and their limitations.

1.4 Alternatives to clinical trials

Evaluating a new intervention requires comparing it with another. This can be done using a randomised clinical trial (RCT), observational study or trial with historical controls (Box 1.1). Although observational studies need to be interpreted carefully with regard to the design features and other influential factors, their results could be consistent with those from an RCT. For example, a review of 20 observational studies indicated that giving a flu vaccine to the elderly could halve the risk of developing respiratory and flu-like symptoms.[6] Practically the same effect was found in a large RCT.[7]

One of the main limitations of observational studies is that the treatment effect could be larger than that found in RCTs or, worse still, a treatment effect is found but RCTs show either no evidence of an effect, or that the intervention is worse. An example of the latter is β-carotene intake and cardiovascular mortality. Combining the results from six observational studies indicated that people with a high β-carotene intake, by eating lots of fruit and vegetables, had a much lower risk of cardiovascular death than those with a low intake (31% reduction in risk).[8] However, combining the results from four randomised trials showed that a high intake might increase the risk by 12%.[8]

Observational (non-randomised) studies

Observational studies may be useful in evaluating treatments with large effects, although there may still be uncertainty over the actual size of the effect. They can be larger than RCTs and therefore provide more evidence on side-effects, particularly uncommon ones. However, when the treatment effect is small or moderate, there are potential design problems associated with observational studies that make it difficult to establish whether a new intervention is truly effective. These are called **confounding** and **bias**.

Several observational studies have examined the effect of a flu vaccine in preventing flu, respiratory disease or death in elderly individuals. Such a study would involve taking a group of people aged over 60 years, then ascertaining whether each subject had had a flu vaccine or not, and which subsequently developed flu or flu-related illnesses. An example is given in Figure 1.1.[9] The chance of developing flu-like illness was lower in the vaccine group than in the unvaccinated group: 21 versus 33%. But did the flu vaccine really work?

The vaccinated group may be people who *chose* to go to their family doctor and request the vaccine, or the doctor or carer recommended it, perhaps on the basis of a perceived increased risk. Unvaccinated people could include those who refused to be vaccinated when offered. It is therefore possible that people who were vaccinated had different lifestyles and characteristics than unvaccinated people, and it is one or more of these factors that partly or wholly explains the lower flu risk, not the effect of the vaccine.

Assume that vitamin C protects against acquiring flu. If people who choose to have the vaccine also happen to eat much more fruit than those who are unvaccinated, then a difference in flu rates would be observed (Table 1.1). The difference of 5 versus 10% could be due to the difference in the proportion of people who ate fruit (80 versus 15%). This is **confounding**. However, if fruit intake had not been measured, it could be incorrectly concluded that the difference in flu rates is due to one group being vaccinated and the other not.

When the association between an intervention (e.g. flu vaccine) and a disorder (e.g. flu) is examined, a spurious relationship could be created through a third factor, called a **confounder** (e.g. eating fruit). A confounder is correlated

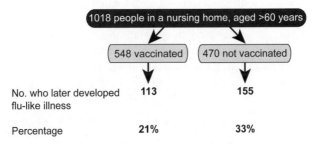

Figure 1.1 Example of an observational study of the flu vaccine.[9]

Table 1.1 Hypothetical observational study of the flu vaccine.

	1000 people aged ≥60 years	
	Vaccinated N = 200	Not vaccinated N = 800
Eat fruit regularly	160 (80%)	120 (15%)
Developed flu 12 months after being vaccinated	10 (5%)	80 (10%)

with both the intervention and the disorder of interest. Confounding factors are often present in observational studies. Even though there are methods of design and analysis that can allow for their effects, there could exist unknown confounders for which no adjustment can be made because they were not measured.

There may also be a **bias**, where the actions of subjects or researchers produce a value of the trial endpoint that is *systematically* under- or over-reported in one trial arm. In the example above, the clinician or carer could deliberately choose fitter people to be vaccinated, believing they would benefit the most. The effect of the vaccine could then be over-estimated, because these particular people may be less likely to acquire the flu than the less fit ones.

Confounding and bias could work together, in that both lead to an under- or over-estimate of the treatment effect, or they could work in opposite directions. It is difficult to separate their effects reliably (Box 1.2). Confounding is sometimes described as a form of bias, since both distort the results. However, it is useful to distinguish them because known confounding factors can be allowed for in a statistical analysis, but it is difficult to do so for bias.

Despite the potential design limitations of observational studies, they can often complement results from randomised trials.[10–14]

Box 1.2 Confounding and bias

- **Confounding** represents the natural relationships between our physical and biochemical characteristics, genetic make-up, and lifestyle and habits that may affect how an individual responds to a treatment. It cannot be removed from a research study, but known confounders can be allowed for in a statistical analysis, and sometimes at the design stage (matched case-control studies).
- **Bias** is usually a design feature of a study that affects how subjects are selected for the study, treated, managed or assessed
- It can be prevented, but human nature often makes this difficult
- It is difficult, sometimes impossible, to allow for bias in a statistical analysis.

Randomisation, within a clinical trial, minimises the effect of confounding and bias on the results

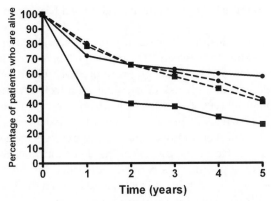

Figure 1.2 Comparison of survival in patients treated with shunt surgery (circles) and medical management (squares). The solid lines are based on a review of five studies, comparing patients treated with surgery at the time of the study, with those treated with medical management in the past. The dashed lines are from a review of eight randomised controlled trials, in which patients were randomly allocated to receive either treatment. The figure is based on information reported in Sacks et al.[15]

Historical (non-randomised) controls

Studies using historical controls may be difficult to interpret because they compare a group of patients treated using one therapy now, with those treated using another therapy in the past. The difference in calendar period is likely to have an effect because it may reflect possible differences in patient characteristics, methods of diagnosis or standards of care. Time would be a confounder. In RCTs, subjects in the trial arms are prospectively followed up simultaneously, so changes over time should not matter. The following example illustrates how using historical controls can give the wrong conclusion.

Patients suffering from cirrhosis with oesophageal varices have dilated sub-mucosal veins in the oesophagus. Figure 1.2 shows the summary results on survival in patients treated with surgery (shunt procedures) or medical management.[15] Survival was substantially better in surgical patients in the fives studies that used historical controls, indicated by a large gap between the solid survival curves. However, the eight RCTs showed no evidence of a benefit; the dashed curves are close together. Survival was clearly poorest in the historical control patients, and this could be due to lower standards of care at that time.

1.5 A randomised trial may not always be the best study design

Although a randomised controlled trial is an appropriate design for most interventions, this is not always the case. When planning a study, initial thought should be given to the disorder of interest, the intervention and any information that could affect either how the study is conducted or the results.

The following example illustrates how a randomised trial could be inferior to another design.

The UK National Health Service study on antenatal Down's syndrome screening was conducted between 1996 and 2000.[16] Screening involves measuring several serum markers in the pregnant mother's blood, which are used to identify those with a high risk of carrying an affected foetus. The study aimed to compare the second trimester Quadruple test (four serum markers measured at 15–19 weeks of pregnancy) with the first trimester Combined test (an ultrasound marker and two other serum markers measured at 10–14 weeks). The main outcome measure was the detection rate: the percentage of Down's syndrome pregnancies correctly identified by the screening test. Women classified as high risk by the test would be offered an invasive diagnostic test to confirm or rule out an affected pregnancy.

At first glance, a randomised trial seems like the obvious design. Pregnant women would be randomly allocated to have either the Combined test or the Quadruple test. The detection rates in the two trial arms would then be compared. However, there are two major limitations with this approach:

Sample size. Preliminary studies suggested a detection rate of 85% for the Combined test and 70% for the Quadruple test. To detect this difference requires a sample size of 95 Down's syndrome pregnancies in each arm. The prevalence in the second trimester is about 1.7 per 1000 (0.0017), so 56 000 women would be needed in each arm (95/0.0017), or 112 000 in total. This would be a very large study that may not be feasible in a reasonable timeframe.

Bias. About 25% of Down's syndrome pregnancies miscarry naturally between the first and second trimesters of pregnancy. In a randomised trial there would be an expected 127 cases seen in the first trimester and 95 in the second trimester. The problem is that the Combined test group would include affected foetuses destined to miscarry, while the Quadruple test group has already had these miscarriages excluded, because a woman allocated to have this test but who miscarried at 12 weeks would clearly not be screened in the second trimester. The comparison of the two screening tests would not be comparing like with like, and it can be shown that the detection rate for the Combined Test would be biased upwards.

A better design is an observational study where both screening tests can be compared in the same woman, which is what happened.[16] Women had an ultrasound during the first trimester and gave a blood sample in both trimesters, but the Combined or Quadruple test markers were not measured or examined until the end of the study (no intervention based on these results); women just received the standard second trimester test according to local policy, the result of which was reported and acted upon. This design avoids the miscarriage bias because only Down's syndrome pregnancies during or after the second trimester were known and included in the analysis. The comparison of the Combined and Quadruple tests was thus based on the same group of pregnancies. Furthermore, because each woman had both tests, a within-person statistical analysis could be performed, and this required only half the number needed compared to a randomised two-arm trial (56 000 instead of 112 000).

1.6 Types of clinical trials

Clinical trials have different objectives. The methods for designing and analysing clinical trials can be applied to experiments on almost any object, for example, animals or cells, as well as humans. They can be broadly categorised into four types (Phase I, II, III or IV), largely depending on the main aim (Box 1.3).

Phase I trials

After a new drug is tested in animal experiments, it is given to humans. Phase I trials are therefore often referred to as 'first in man' studies. They are used to examine the pharmacological actions of the new drug (i.e. how

---

Box 1.3 Types of trials

Phase I

- First time a new drug or regimen is tested on humans
- Few participants (say <30)
- Primary aims are to find a dose with an acceptable level of safety, and examine the biological and pharmacological effects

Phase II

- Not too large (say 30–70 people)
- Aim is to obtain a *preliminary* estimate of efficacy
- Not designed to determine whether a new treatment works
- Produces data in each of the trial arms, that could be used to design a phase III trial

Phase III

- Must be randomised and with a comparison (control) group
- Relatively large (usually several hundred or thousand people)
- Aim is to provide a *definitive* answer on whether a new treatment is better than the control group, or is similarly effective but there are other advantages

Phase IV

- Relatively large (usually several hundred or thousand people)
- Used to continue to monitor efficacy and safety in the population once the new treatment has been adopted into routine practice.

it is processed in the body), but also to find a dose level that has acceptable side-effects. They may provide early evidence on effectiveness.

Phase I trials are typically small, often less than 30 individuals, and based on healthy volunteers. An exception may be in trials in specialties where the intervention is expected to have side effects, so it is inappropriate to give it to healthy people, but rather those who already have the disorder of interest (e.g. cancer). Subjects are closely monitored. Phase I studies may be conducted in a short space of time, with few recruiting centres, depending on how common the disease is and the type of intervention. There may be several phase I trials, and if the results are favourable, they are used to design a phase II trial. Many new drugs are not investigated further.

Phase II trials

The aim of a phase II study is to obtain a preliminary assessment of efficacy in a group of subjects that is not large, say less than 100 and often around 50. These trials can be conducted relatively quickly, without spending too many resources (participants, time and money) on something that may not work. As in phase I studies, participants are closely monitored for safety.

A phase II study could have several new treatments to examine. There could also be a control arm in which subjects are given standard therapy, because the disease of interest is relatively uncommon, so there is uncertainty over the effect of the standard therapy. If the results are positive, the data in each arm are used to design a randomised phase III trial, for example estimating sample size. When there is more than one intervention, it is best, though not absolutely necessary, to randomise subjects to the trial groups. The advantages of randomising are given on page 12. A randomised phase II study could also provide information on the feasibility of a subsequent phase III trial, such as how willing subjects are to be randomised.

Phase III trials

A phase III trial is commonly referred to as a **randomised controlled trial (RCT)**. Subjects must be **randomly allocated** to the intervention groups, and there must be a **control (comparison)**. The aim is to provide a definitive answer on whether a new intervention is better than the control, or sometimes whether they have a similar effect. Sometimes, there are more than two new interventions. Phase III studies are often large, involving several hundred or thousand people. Results should be precise and robust enough to persuade health professionals to change practice. The larger the trial, the more reliable the conclusions. The size of these trials, and the need for several recruiting centres, mean that they can take several years to complete.

There is sometimes a misunderstanding that a randomised phase II trial is a quick randomised phase III trial, but they have quite different purposes. A randomised phase II study is not usually designed for a direct statistical comparison of the trial endpoint between the two interventions, and this is reflected in the smaller sample size. Therefore, the results cannot be used to make a reliable conclusion on whether the new intervention is better.

However, a phase III trial is designed for a direct comparison, allowing a full evaluation of the new intervention and, usually, a definitive conclusion.[#]

Phase III trials should be designed and conducted to a high standard, with precise quantitative results on efficacy and safety. This can be particularly important for pharmaceutical companies who wish to obtain a marketing licence from a regulatory agency for a new drug or medical device, which normally requires extensive data before a licence is granted. Trials used in this way can be referred to as **pivotal trials**.

Phase IV trials

These are sometimes referred to as **post-marketing** or **surveillance** studies. Once a new treatment has been evaluated using a phase III trial and adopted into clinical practice, some organisations (usually the pharmaceutical industry) continue to monitor the efficacy and safety of the new intervention. Because several thousand people could be included, phase IV studies may be useful in identifying uncommon adverse effects not seen in the preceding phase III trials. They are also based on subjects in the general target population, rather than the selected group of subjects who agree to participate in a phase III trial. However, phase IV studies are not as common as the other trial types, particularly in the academic or public sector. Comparisons can sometimes only be made with historical controls or groups of people (non-users of the new drug) who are likely to have different characteristics. Because of this, phase IV studies are not discussed in further detail in this book, though the methods of analysis for phase III trials can be used.

1.7 Four key design features

The study population of all types of clinical trials must be defined by the **inclusion and exclusion criteria**. The strength of randomised phase II and III trials comes from three further design features: **control**, **randomisation** and **blinding**.

Inclusion and exclusion criteria

It is necessary to specify which participants are recruited. This is done using a set of **inclusion and exclusion** criteria (or **eligibility list**), which each subject has to fulfil before entry. Every trial will have its own criteria depending on the objectives, and this may include an age range, having no serious co-morbid conditions, the ability to obtain consent, and that subjects have not previously taken the trial treatment. They should have unambiguous definitions to make recruiting subjects easier.

[#]Some researchers design a study as if it were a phase III trial, but using a one-sided test with a permissive level of statistical significance $\geq 10\%$ (see Chapter 5) and usually a surrogate endpoint (see Chapter 2). It is however referred to as a randomised phase II trial. The description of randomised phase II studies given in this book is the one preferred here.

Table 1.2 Hypothetical example of inclusion and exclusion criteria for a trial of a new drug for preventing stroke.

Narrow set of criteria	
Inclusion	*Exclusion*
Male	History of heart disease or stroke
Age 50 to 55 years	History of cancer
Never-smoker	Female
	Ex and current smokers
	Unable to give informed consent
	Family history of heart disease
	Average alcohol intake <2 units per day

Wide set of criteria	
Inclusion	*Exclusion*
Male or female	Unable to give informed consent
Age 45 to 85 years	

Determining the eligibility criteria necessitates balancing the advantages and disadvantages of having a highly selected group against those associated with including a wide variety of subjects. Having many criteria which are narrow (Table 1.2), produces a group in which there should be relatively little variability. Subjects are more likely to respond to the treatment in a similar manner, and this makes it easier to detect an effect if it exists, especially if the effect is small or moderate. However, the trial results may only apply to a small proportion of the population, and so may not be easily generalisable. A trial with few criteria, that are wide (Table 1.2), will have a more general application, but the amount of variability is expected to be high. This could make it more difficult to show that the treatment is effective. When there is much variability, sometimes only large effects can be detected easily.

Control group

The outcome of subjects given the new intervention is always compared with that in a group who are not receiving the new intervention. A **control** group normally receives the current standard of care, no intervention or placebo (see Blinding below). Treatment effects from randomised trials are therefore always relative. The choice of the control intervention depends on the availability of alternative treatments. When an established treatment exists, it is unethical to give a placebo instead because this deprives some subjects of a known health benefit.

Randomisation

In order to attribute a difference in outcome between two trial arms to the new treatment being tested, the characteristics of people should be similar between the groups. In the hypothetical example of the flu vaccine (Table 1.1),

---

Box 1.4 Randomisation

• Randomly allocating subjects produces groups that are as similar as possible with regard to all characteristics except the trial interventions

• The only systematic difference between the two arms should be the treatment given

• Therefore, any differences in results observed at the end of the trial should be due to the effect of the new treatment, and not to any other factors (or differences in characteristics have not spuriously produced a treatment effect, when the aim is to show that the interventions have a similar effect).

---

the difference in flu risk at the end of the trial could be due to the difference in those who ate fruit regularly (**confounding**), not the vaccine. Randomly allocating patients to the trial arms means that any difference in outcome at the end of the trial should be due to the new treatment being tested, and not any other factor (Box 1.4).

Randomisation is a process for allocating subjects between the different trial interventions. Each subject has the same chance of being allocated to any group, which ensures similarity in characteristics between the arms. This minimises the effect of both known and unknown confounders, and thus has a distinct advantage over observational studies in which statistical adjustments can only be made for known confounders. Although randomisation is designed to produce groups with similar characteristics, there will always be small differences because of chance variation. Randomisation cannot produce *identical* groups.

Randomisation also minimises **bias**. If either the researcher or trial subject is allowed to decide which intervention is allocated, then subjects with a certain characteristic, for example, those who are younger or with less severe disease, could be over-represented in one of the trial arms. This could produce a bias which makes the new intervention look effective when it really is not, or over-estimate the treatment effect. **Selection bias** can occur if a choosing a particular subject for the trial is influenced by knowing the next treatment allocation. **Allocation bias** involves giving the trial treatment that the clinician or subject feels might be most beneficial. Sometimes, the researcher has access to the list of randomisations from which the next allocation can be seen, possibly creating allocation bias. This can be avoided if randomisation is done through a central office (for example, a clinical trials unit) or a computer system, because the researcher has no control over either process (called **allocation concealment**).

Blinding

The randomisation process minimises the potential for bias, but the benefit could be greater if the trial intervention given to each subject is concealed. Subjects or researchers may have expectations associated with a particular treatment, and knowing which was given can create bias. This can affect how people respond to treatment, or how the researcher manages or assesses the subject. In subjects, this bias is specifically referred to as the **placebo effect**. Humans have a remarkable psychological ability to affect their own health status. The effect of any of these biases could result in subjects receiving the new intervention appearing to do better than those on the control treatment, but the difference is not really due to the action of the new treatment.

Clinical trials are described as **double-blind** if neither the subject nor any-one involved in giving the treatment, or managing or assessing the subject, is aware of which treatment was given. In **single-blind** trials, usually only the subject is blind to the treatment they have received (see also page 61).

A placebo has no known active component. It is often referred to as a 'sugar pill' because many treatment trials involve swallowing tablets. How-ever, a placebo could also be a saline injection, a sham surgical procedure, sham medical device or any other intervention that is meant to resemble the test intervention, but has no known effect on the disease of interest, and no adverse effect. A recent example was based on patients with osteoarthritis of the knee who often undergo surgery (arthroscopic lavage or débridement). There were more than 650 000 procedures each year in the USA around 2002. However, a randomised trial,[17] comparing these two surgical procedures with sham surgery (skin incision to the knee) provided no evidence that these pro-cedures reduced knee pain. This trial was justified on the basis that patients in uncontrolled studies reported less pain after having the procedure despite there being no clear biological reason for this.

Using placebos needs to be fully justified in any clinical trial. While there are some arguments against placebos such as sham surgery, these trials can provide valuable evidence on the effectiveness of a new intervention. They can be conducted as long as there is ethical approval, and patients are fully aware that they may be assigned to the sham group.

When it is not possible to conceal the trial interventions, an outcome mea-sure that does not depend on the personal opinion of the subject or researcher is best. For example, in a trial evaluating hypnotherapy for smoking cessation, a subjective measure would be to ask the subjects if they stopped smoking at, say, 1 year. However, there could be some continuing smokers who misreport their smoking status. An objective endpoint would be to measure serum or urinary cotinine, as a marker of current smoking status, because this is specific to tobacco smoke inhalation, and so less prone to bias than a questionnaire on self-reported habits.

1.8 Small trials

Trials with a small number of subjects can be quick to conduct with regard to enrolling patients, performing biochemical analyses, or asking subjects to complete study questionnaires. A possible advantage is, therefore, that the research question could be examined in a relatively short space of time. Fur-thermore, small studies are usually only conducted across a few centres, so obtaining all ethical and institutional approvals should be quicker compared to large multi-centre studies.

It is often useful to examine a new intervention in a few subjects first (as in a phase II trial). This avoids spending too many resources, such as subjects, time and financial costs, on looking for a treatment effect when there really is none. However, if a positive result is found it is important to make clear in the conclusions that a larger confirmatory study is needed.

The main limitation of small trials is in interpreting their results, in particular confidence intervals and p-values (Chapter 7). They can often produce false-positive results or over-estimate the magnitude of the treatment benefit. Overly small trials may yield results that are too unreliable and therefore uninformative. While there is nothing wrong with conducting well-designed small studies, they must be interpreted carefully, without making strong conclusions.

1.9 Summary points

• Clinical trials are essential for evaluating new methods of disease detection, prevention and treatment
• Observational studies can provide useful supporting evidence on the effectiveness of an intervention
• Clinical trials, especially when randomised, are considered to provide the strongest evidence
• Randomisation minimises the effect of confounding and bias, and blinding further reduces the potential for bias.

Key design features of clinical trials

1. Inclusion and exclusion criteria
2. Controlled (comparison/control arm)
3. Randomisation
4. Blinding (using placebo)

References

1. Laine C, Horton R, DeAngelis CD *et al*. Clinical Trial Registration: Looking Back and Moving Ahead. *Ann Intern Med* 2007; **147(4)**:275–277.
2. World Health Organization. International Clinical Trials Registry Platform. http://www.who.int/ictrp/about/details/en/index.html
3. http://www.jameslindlibrary.org/trial_records/17th_18th_Century/lind/lind_tp.html
4. Hróbjartsson A, Gøtzsche PC, Gluud C. The controlled clinical trial turns 100 years: Fibiger's trial of serum treatment of diphtheria. *BMJ* 1998; **317**:1243–1245.

5. Medical Research Council. Streptomycin treatment of pulmonary tuberculosis. *BMJ* 1948; **2**:769–782.

6. Gross PA, Hermogenes H, Sacks HS, Lau J, Levandowski RA. The efficacy of influenza vaccine in elderly persons. *Ann Intern Med* 1995; **123**:518–527.

7. Govaert TME, Thijs CTMCN, Masurel N *et al.* The efficacy of influenza vaccination in elderly individuals. *JAMA* 1994; **272**(21):1661–1665.

8. Egger M, Schneider M, Davey Smith G. Meta-analysis: spurious precision? Meta-analysis of observational studies. *BMJ* 1998; **316**:140–144.

9. Patriarca PA, Weber JA, Parker RA *et al.* Efficacy of influenza vaccine in nursing homes. Reduction in illness and complications during an influenza A (H3N2) epidemic. *JAMA* 1985; **253**:1136–1139.

10. Benson K, Hartz AJ. A comparison of observational studies and randomised controlled trials. *N Eng J Med* 2000; **342**:1878–1886.

11. Concato J, Shah N, Horwitz RI. Randomized controlled trials, observational studies, and the hierarchy of research designs. *N Eng J Med* 2000; **342**:1887–1892.

12. Pocock SJ, Elbourne DR. Randomized trials or observational tribulations? *N Eng J Med* 2000; **342**:1907–1909.

13. Collins R, MacMahon S. Reliable assessment of the effects of treatment on mortality and major morbidity, I: clinical trials. *The Lancet* 2001; **357**:373–380.

14. MacMahon S, Collins R. Reliable assessment of the effects of treatment on mortality and major morbidity, II: observational studies. *The Lancet* 2001; **357**:455–462.

15. Sacks H, Chalmers TC, Smith H. Randomized versus historical controls for clinical trials. *Am J Med* 1982; **72**:233–240.

16. Wald NJ, Rodeck CH, Hackshaw AK *et al.* First and second trimester antenatal screening for Down's syndrome: the results of the Serum, Urine and Ultrasound Screening Study (SURUSS). *Health Technology Assessment* 2003; **7**(11).

17. Moseley JB, O'Malley K, Petersen NJ *et al.* A Controlled Trial of Arthroscopic Surgery for Osteoarthritis of the Knee. *N Eng J Med* 2002; **347**(2):81–88.

CHAPTER 2

Types of outcome measures and understanding them

When statin therapy was first shown to be an effective treatment for preventing heart disease, it would not have been sufficient just to say 'statins are effective'. This statement is unclear. What does 'effective' actually mean? It could be a reduction in the chance of having a first coronary event, a reduction in the chance of having a subsequent coronary event in those who have already suffered one, a reduction in serum cholesterol, or a reduction in the chance of dying. Each of these is an **outcome measure** or **endpoint**, and when they are clearly defined they contribute not only to the appropriate design of a clinical trial, but also to an easier and clearer interpretation of the results.

2.1 'True' versus surrogate outcome measures

Some outcome measures have an obvious and direct clinical relevance to participants, for example, whether they:
- Live or die
- Develop a disorder or not
- Recover from a disease or not
- Change their lifestyle or habits (e.g. stopped smoking)
- Have a change in body weight

A clear impact of statins is evident in a clinical trial using the outcome measure 'coronary event or no coronary event'. Death, occurrence of a disease, and other similar measures are sometimes referred to as **'true' outcomes** or **endpoints**. For several disorders there is the concept of a **surrogate endpoint**.[1-3] These are measures that do not often have an obvious impact that subjects are able to identify. They are usually assumed to be a precursor to the true outcome, i.e. they lie along the causal pathway. Surrogate markers can be a blood measurement, or examined by medical imaging tests (Box 2.1).

Sometimes, a trial would have to be impractically large, or take many years to conduct, because a true endpoint would have too few events to allow a reliable evaluation of the intervention. A surrogate marker is attractive because

A concise guide to clinical trials, First edition. By A. Hackshaw. Published 2009 by Blackwell Publishing, ISBN: 978-1-4051-6774-1.

Box 2.1 Examples of true and surrogate trial endpoints

Surrogate endpoint	True endpoint
Cholesterol level	Heart attack or death from heart attack
Blood pressure	Stroke or death from stroke
Tumour response (partial or complete remission of tumour)	Survival
Time to cancer progression	Survival
Tooth pocket depth or attachment level	Tooth loss (in periodontitis)
CD4 count	Death from AIDS
Total brain volume	Progression of Alzheimer's disease
Hippocampal volume	Progression of Alzheimer's disease
Loss of dopaminergic neurons	Progression of Parkinson's disease
Intra-ocular pressure	Glaucoma

---

there are more events, possibly in a shorter space of time, so trials could be conducted quicker or with fewer subjects, thus saving resources. Using a surrogate might be the only feasible option to evaluate a new potential treatment. The surrogate and true endpoints need to be closely correlated: a change in the surrogate outcome measure now is likely to produce a change in a more clinically important outcome, such as death or prevention of a disorder, later. Studies that show this **validate** the surrogate marker.

Statin therapy reduces serum cholesterol levels, which in turn reduces the risk of a heart attack. Cholesterol is therefore an accepted surrogate endpoint when examining some therapies for coronary heart disease; a claim in benefit of a new drug could come from a randomised trial in which cholesterol levels have been significantly reduced. In other diseases, it is difficult to find good surrogates. For example, tumour response[#] does not correlate well with survival in several cancers, such as advanced breast cancer. Therefore, while tumour response can provide useful information on the biological course of a cancer, and be used in phase I or II studies, it would not be the main endpoint in a phase III trial evaluating a new therapy.

It is essential to consider whether the measure used in a particular study is meaningful and appropriate for addressing the primary objectives. There is sometimes a danger that the true endpoint is not investigated thoroughly,

---

[#] Defined as a partial and/or complete response, in which the tumour has substantially reduced in size or disappeared clinically.

and it can be hard to arrive at firm conclusions on the effectiveness of a new treatment when the evidence is based solely on surrogate measures. When evaluating a new drug or medical device, it might be useful to check with the regulatory authority that a proposed surrogate marker is acceptable. While surrogate measures are commonly investigated in early phase trials (phase I and II), their use in confirmatory phase III trials needs careful consideration and validation.

2.2 Types of outcomes

Outcome measures fall into two basic categories: **counting people** and **taking measurements on people**. There is a special case of 'taking measurements' that is based on **time-to-event data**. It is useful to distinguish between them because it helps to define the trial objectives, and methods of sample size calculation and statistical analysis. First, the **unit of interest** is determined, usually a person. Second, consider what will be done to the unit of interest. The outcome measure will involve either **counting** how many people have a particular characteristic (i.e. put them into mutually exclusive groups, such as 'dead' or 'alive'), or **taking measurements** on them. In some situations, taking a measurement on someone involves counting something, but the unit of interest is still a person. Box 2.2 shows examples of outcome measures.

Having measured the endpoint for each trial subject it is necessary to summarise the data in a form that can be readily communicated to others.

Box 2.2 Examples of outcome measures when the unit of interest is a person

Counting people (binary or categorical data)

    Dead or alive
    Admitted to hospital (yes or no)
    Suffered a first heart attack (yes or no)
    Recovered from disease (yes or no)
    Severity of disease (mild, moderate, severe)
    Ability to perform household duties (none, a little, some, moderate, high)

Taking measurements on people (continuous data)

    Blood pressure
    Body weight
    Cholesterol level
    Size of tumour
    White blood cell count
    Number of days in hospital
    Number of units of alcohol intake per week

Further details can be found in books on medical statistics (see reading list on page 203).

Types of outcome measures

After defining the health outcome for a trial, what is to be done to the unit of interest, i.e. people?
- Count people, i.e. how many have the health outcome of interest
- Take measurements on people
- Time-to-event measures.

2.3 Counting people

This type of outcome measure is easily summarised by calculating the **percentage** or **proportion**. For example, the effect of a flu vaccine can be examined by counting how many developed flu in the vaccinated group, and dividing this number by the total number of patients in that group. This proportion (or percentage) is the **risk**, i.e. the risk of developing flu if vaccinated. The same calculation is made in the unvaccinated group, i.e. the risk of developing flu if not vaccinated. In Figure 1.1 (page 5), the two risks are 21 and 33%. The word 'risk' implies something negative, but it could be used for any outcome that involves counting people, for example, the risk of being alive after 5 years.

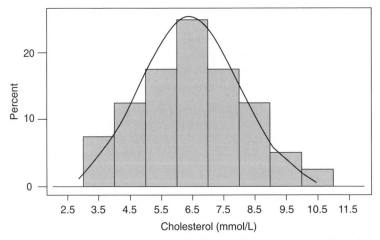

Figure 2.1 Histogram of the cholesterol values in 40 men, with a superimposed Normal distribution curve.

2.4 Taking measurements on people

This type of outcome measure will vary between people. Consider the following cholesterol levels (mmol/L) for 40 healthy men, all aged 45 years (ranked in order of size):

3.6	3.8	3.9	4.1	4.2	4.5	4.5	4.8	5.1	5.3
5.4	5.4	5.6	5.8	5.9	6.0	6.1	6.1	6.2	6.3
6.4	6.5	6.6	6.8	6.9	7.1	7.2	7.2	7.3	7.4
7.5	7.7	8.0	8.1	8.1	8.2	8.3	9.0	9.1	10.0

These data are summarised by two parameters: the 'average' level and a measure of spread or variability. The average, often referred to as a measure of central tendency, can be described by either the **mean** or **median**. It is where the middle of the distribution lies. The mean is more commonly reported and often taken to be the same as the average. Another measure of average is the **mode** – the most frequently occurring value – but there are few instances where this is the best summary measure.

The mean is the sum of all the values divided by the number of observations. In the example above, the mean is $256/40 = 6.4$ mmol/L. The median is the value that has half the observations above it and half below. In the example, it is halfway between the 20th and 21st values; median $= (6.3 + 6.4)/2 = 6.35$ mmol/L.

One measure of spread is the **standard deviation** (Box 2.3). It quantifies the amount of variability in a group of people, i.e. how much the data spreads about from the mean. It is calculated as:

$$\sqrt{\frac{\text{Sum of (the distances of each data point from the mean})^2}{(\text{Number of data values} - 1)}}$$

In the example, the standard deviation is 1.57 mmol/L: the cholesterol levels differ from the mean value of 6.4 by, on average, 1.57 mmol/L.

Another measure of spread is **the interquartile range**. This is the difference between the 25th centile (the value that has a quarter of the data below it and

---

Box 2.3 Illustration of standard deviation for five values

Cholesterol (mmol/L)	4.5	4.9	5.5	5.7	6.2
Difference from the mean (5.36)	−0.86	−0.46	+0.14	+0.34	+0.84

Sum of the differences = 0

So square the differences	0.74	0.21	0.02	0.12	0.70

Sum of the square differences = 1.79
Divide by number of observations minus 1 = $1.79/(5 - 1) = 0.457$
Take the square root to get standard deviation $= \sqrt{0.457} = 0.67$ mmol/L
on the original scale

Cholesterol (mmol/L)	Number of men	Percentage
3.0–3.9	3	7.5
4.0–4.9	5	12.5
5.0–5.9	7	17.5
6.0–6.9	10	25.0
7.0–7.9	7	17.5
8.0–8.9	5	12.5
9.0–9.9	2	5.0
10.0–10.9	1	2.5
Total	40	100.0

Table 2.1 Frequency distribution of cholesterol levels of a sample of 40 men (page 21).

three-quarters above it) and the 75th centile (the value that has three-quarters of the data below it and a quarter above it). In the example, there are 40 observations so the 25th centile is between the 10th and 11th data points (i.e. 5.32 mmol/L) and the 75th centile is between the 30th and 31st data points (i.e. 7.47 mmol/L).[#] The interquartile range is therefore $7.47 - 5.32 = 2.15$ mmol/L. Sometimes, the actual 25th and 75th centiles are presented instead of the interquartile range.

Deciding which measures of average and spread to use depends on whether the distribution is symmetric or not. To help determine this, the data is grouped into categories of cholesterol levels and the **frequency distribution** is examined (Table 2.1). These proportions are used to create a **histogram** (the shaded boxes in Figure 2.1). The shape is reasonably symmetric, indicating that the distribution is **Gaussian** or **Normal** ('N' is in capital letters to avoid confusion with the usual definition of the word normal, which can indicate people without disease). This is more easily visualised by drawing a curve around the histogram (Figure 2.1), which is said to be bell-shaped.

When data are Normally distributed, the mean and median are similar. The preferred measures of average and spread are the mean and standard deviation, because they have useful mathematical properties which underlie many statistical methods used to analyse this type of data. When the data are not Normally distributed, the median and interquartile range are better measures. To understand why, consider the outcome measure *'number of days in hospital'* for 20 patients. The histogram is given in Figure 2.2. It is clear that the distribution is not symmetric. It is **skewed to the right** (this is where the tail of the data is). When most of the data are towards the right, the distribution is said to be **skewed to the left**.

[#]The 25th centile is the point at $(n + 1)/4$, i.e. the 10.25th observation. This is between the 10th and 11th value, i.e. 5.3 and 5.4, and found by adding $0.25 \times$ difference between these two observations (0.1) to 5.3. So the 25th centile is $5.3 + 0.025 = 5.325$. A similar calculation is made to obtain the 75th centile.

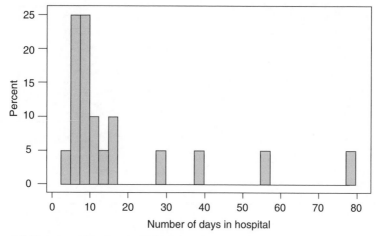

Figure 2.2 Histogram of the length of hospital stay for 20 patients.

The summary statistics that describe this data are:

Mean = 17 days   Standard deviation = 19 days
Median = 9 days   Interquartile range = 8 days

The middle of the data, and spread, are better represented by the median and interquartile range. The mean and standard deviation are heavily influenced by the few very high values.

When data are skewed it is sometimes possible to **transform** it, usually by taking **logarithms** or the **square root**. Many biological measurements only have a Normal (symmetric) distribution after the logarithm is taken, so using the log of the values would produce a histogram that has a similar shape to that in Figure 2.1. The mean is calculated using the log of the values, and the result is back-transformed to the original scale, though this cannot be done with standard deviation. For example, if the mean of the transformed values is 0.81, using log to the base 10, the calculation $10^{0.81} = 6.5$ produces the mean value on the original scale. This is called a **geometric mean**. Sometimes no transformation is possible that will turn a skewed distribution into a Normal one. In these situations, the median and interquartile range should be used.

A **probability** (or **centile**) **plot**[#] can be used to determine whether data is Normally distributed or not. Many statistical software packages can provide this. Figure 2.3 is an example using the 40 cholesterol measurements above. If the observations lie *reasonably* along a straight line, the data are Normally distributed. Another simple check is to examine whether the mean ± 2 ×

[#]Textbooks listed on page 203 can provide a technical description of how the plot is obtained, but what is useful here is how to interpret it.

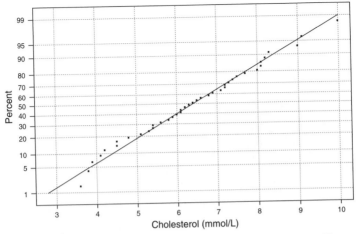

Figure 2.3 Normal probability plot for the 40 cholesterol measurements on page 22.

standard deviation produces sensible numbers. In the example from Figure 2.3, this would be 17 days $\pm(2 \times 19)$: the lower limit of -21 days is implausible.

2.5 Time-to-event data

A specific category of 'taking measurements on people' involves examining the time taken until an event has occurred, based on the difference between two calendar dates. An event could be defined in many ways, and one of the simplest and most commonly used is 'death', hence the term **survival analysis** which is applied to this type of data. This definition of an event is used in this section, but others are given in Section 2.6. In the following seven subjects, the endpoint is 'time from randomisation until death (in years)', and all have died:

4.5   6.1   6.7   8.3   9.1   9.4   10.0

The mean (7.7 years) or median (8.3 years) are easily calculated. In another group of nine subjects, not all have died at the time of statistical analysis:

2.7   2.9   3.3   4.7   5.1   6.8   7.2   7.8   9.1
dead dead alive dead alive alive dead dead alive

The mean or median cannot be calculated in the usual way, until all the subjects have died, which could take many years, and it is incorrect to ignore those still alive because the summary measure would be biased downward. An alternative is to obtain the survival rate at, say, 3 years. In the example, 2 people died before 3 years and 7 lived beyond, so the 3-year survival rate is $7/9 = 78\%$. This is simply an example of 'counting people'. However, every subject needs to be followed up for at least 3 years, unless they died beforehand, and the outcome (dead or alive) must be known at that point for all of them. In many studies this is not possible, particularly with long follow up, because contact is lost with some subjects. This approach also ignores the length of time before a subject dies.

In 1958 a statistical method was developed that changed the way this type of data was displayed and analysed.[4] In the example above, the time-to-event variable is treated as 'time from randomisation until death or last known to be alive' (instead of 'time from randomisation until death'), and there is another variable with the values 0 or 1 to indicate 'still alive' or 'dead'. A subject who is still alive, or last known to be alive at a certain date, is said to be **censored**. The two variables are used in a **life-table** from which it is possible to construct a **Kaplan–Meier plot**. This approach uses the last available information on every subject and how long he/she has lived for, or has been in the study. It is therefore less of a concern if contact with some subjects was lost because having the date when they were last known to be alive still provides information.

Table 2.2 and Figure 2.4 are based on the group of nine subjects above. The plot looks like a series of steps. Every time a subjects dies, the step drops down (the first drop is at 2.7 years). When subjects are censored, four in the example, they contribute no further information to the analysis after that date. In large studies with many deaths, the plot looks smoother.

It is possible to estimate survival rates at specific time points, and the median survival. For the 5-year survival rate, a vertical line is drawn on the x-axis at '5' and the corresponding y-axis value is taken when the line hits the curve: 65% (Figure 2.4). The median is the time at which half the subjects have died. A horizontal line is drawn on the y-axis at '50%' and the corresponding x-axis value is taken when the line hits the curve: 7.2 years. These estimates are more accurately obtained from the life-table (Table 2.2).

Table 2.2 Life-table for the survival data of nine patients on page 24.

Time since randomisation (years)	Censored (0 = yes, 1 = dead)	Number of patients at risk	Percentage alive (survival rate %)
0	–	9	100
2.7	1	9	89
2.9	1	8	78
3.3	0	7	78
4.7	1	6	65
5.1	0	5	65
6.8	0	4	65
7.2	1	3	43
7.8	1	2	22
9.1	0	1	22

• To obtain the 5-year survival rate from the table it is necessary to ascertain whether there is a value at exactly 5 years. Because there is not, the closest value from below is taken, i.e. at 4.7 years: 5-year survival rate is 65%.
• The median survival is the point at which 50% of patients are alive. The closest value from below is 43%, so the median is 7.2 years.

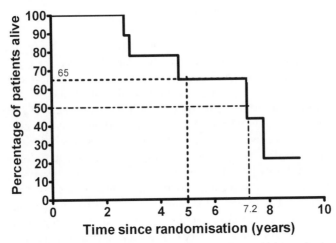

Figure 2.4 Kaplan–Meier plot of the survival data for nine patients, which can also be used to estimate survival rates and median survival.

When some subjects are censored, i.e. not all have died, the Kaplan–Meier median survival is not the same as finding the median from a ranked list of numbers (as in the example on page 21). They are only identical when every subject has died, which is rare in trials. The median is used instead of the mean, because time-to-event data often has a skewed distribution.

The Kaplan–Meier plot starts off with every subject alive at time zero; this is the most common form in the literature. This type of plot is useful when deaths tend to occur early on. However, it is possible to have a plot in which no subject has died at time zero. Figure 2.5 uses the same data as in Figure 2.4, but the death (i.e. event) rate instead of the survival rate is shown on the y-axis

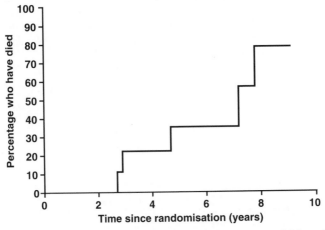

Figure 2.5 Kaplan–Meier plot of the survival data for nine patients on page 24, based on cumulative risk.

(100 minus the fourth column in Table 2.2). This type of plot may be more informative when deaths tend to occur later on. A curve based on the survival rate has to start at 100% at time zero, but because the y-axis for the death rate starts at zero, the upper limit can be chosen, allowing differences between two treatments to be seen more clearly.

Different types of time-to-event outcome measures

In the section above, the 'event' in the time-to-event data is 'death'; called **overall survival** because it relates to death from any cause. The methods can apply to any endpoint that involves measuring the time until a specified event has occurred, for example, time from entry to a trial until the occurrence or recurrence of a disorder, such as severe exacerbation of asthma, or any change in health status, such as time until hospital discharge. The 'event' should be clearly specified. Box 2.4 shows commonly used time-to-event endpoints.

Overall survival is simple because it only requires the date of death. Cause-specific survival requires, in addition, accurate confirmation of cause of death (such as pathology records), which is not always available or reliably recorded. Also, cause-specific survival means that deaths from causes other than that of interest are not counted as an event (they are censored). This may be inappropriate when the treatment has serious side-effects. A new therapy may reduce the lung cancer death rate, but increase the risk of dying from treatment-related side-effects, for example, cardiovascular disease. Here, overall survival is probably more appropriate.

When an event is disease incidence,[#] recurrence or progression, the date when this occurs is required. However, obtaining accurate dates is difficult unless subjects are examined regularly. The date is usually when the disease was first discovered. This is either the date when the subject was due to have one of the regular examinations specified in the trial protocol (see page 161), or after the subject developed symptoms and received clinical confirmation. Subjects in the trial arms should therefore have their regular examinations at a similar time. If, for example, Group A have their examinations earlier than Group B, this could bias the endpoint in favour of Group B (Figure 2.6).

When the measure is based on two or more event types and a subject could have both events, such as disease occurrence followed by death, it is usual to consider only the date of the first event in the analysis. This is because the patient may be managed differently afterwards: the trial treatment changes or stops, non-trial therapies are given, or patients may be given the treatment from the other trial arm. When this occurs, it is difficult dealing with subsequent events, and how to attribute differences in the endpoint to the trial treatments. Unlike overall survival, disease-, progression- or event-free survival are unaffected by subsequent treatments because only the first event matters in the analysis.

[#]The first time the subject develops the disease of interest.

Box 2.4 Time-to-event outcome measures in trials

Endpoint	An event is defined as follows. All other subjects are censored	Comments
Overall survival	Death from any cause	Easily defined
		May mask the effects of an intervention if it only affects a specific disease
Disease-free survival	First recurrence of the disease Death from any cause	Useful when patients are thought to be free from disease after treatment, so patients have a good prognosis Needs date of recurrence
Event-free survival	First recurrence of the disease First occurrence of other specified diseases Death from any cause	Similar to disease-free survival
Progression-free survival	First sign of disease progression Death from any cause	Useful for advanced disease, where patients have not been 'cured' after treatment, and are expected to get worse in the near future Needs date of progression
Disease (or cause)-specific survival	Death from the disease of interest	Useful when examining interventions that are not expected to have an effect on any disease apart from the one of interest Needs accurate recording and confirmation of cause of death Assumes treatment is not associated with deaths from other causes
Time-to-treatment failure	First sign of disease progression Death from any cause Stopped treatment	Similar to progression-free survival

Recurrence: there was no clinical evidence of the disease shortly after treatment, but the disease returned later on.
Progression (or relapse): the patient still had the disease after treatment, but it got worse later.
Disease and event-free survival may be used interchangeably, so it is useful to be clear about the precise definition.

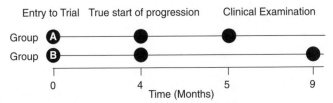

Figure 2.6 Two hypothetical patients from Groups A and B, whose disease has the same biological course but with different dates of first clinical examination.
Recorded time to progression is: 5 months for patient in Group A and 9 months for patient in Group B. It would falsely appear that Group B has a greater benefit.

2.6 Summary points

- Trials should have clearly defined outcome measures (endpoints)
- Surrogate endpoints should be closely correlated with 'true' endpoints, and have been validated, especially if they are used as the main trial endpoint
- Outcome measures could involve 'counting people', 'taking measurements on people' or 'time-to-event' data
- Counting people: data are summarised by a percentage or proportion (risk)
- Taking measurements on people: data are summarised by average and spread (mean and standard deviation if the data are Normally distributed, median and interquartile range if the data are skewed)
- Time-to-event data: when not all patients have had the event of interest: the data can be summarised using a Kaplan–Meier plot, median value, or survival or event-rate at a specific time point.

References

1. Katz R. Biomarkers and surrogate markers: an FDA perspective. *NeuroRx: J Am Soc Exp NeuroTherap* 2004; **1**:189–195.
2. Temple R. Are surrogate markers adequate to assess cardiovascular disease drugs? *JAMA* 1999; **282(8)**:790–795.
3. Guidance for industry: clinical trial endpoints for the approval of cancer drugs and biologics. http://www.fda.gov/CbER/gdlns/clintrialend.htm.
4. Kaplan EL, Meier P. Nonparametric estimation from incomplete observations. *J Am Stat Assoc* 1958; **53**:457–481.

CHAPTER 3

Design and analysis of phase I trials

Phase I trials, often referred to as 'first in man' studies, are conducted to examine the biological and pharmacological actions of a new treatment (usually a new drug), and its side-effects. They are almost always preceded by several *in vitro* studies and studies in mammals. A more detailed discussion of the design, conduct and analysis of phase I trials is found in the references.[1-4]

3.1 Design

Phase I studies are exploratory, and they usually aim to determine a sufficiently safe dose. They involve giving a certain dose to a few subjects, and if tolerable, the next group receive a higher dose. This continues until the administered dose is associated with an unacceptable level of side-effects. This is not the same as trying to find the most effective (optimal) dose, which is the objective of phase II and III trials. Although there needs to be a small number of subjects in each dose group, the study should provide enough information on safety and efficacy to determine whether a new drug should be investigated further. This can be a difficult balance to achieve. Few trials have formal methods for estimating the total sample size because the number of subjects recruited will largely depend on the design employed and how many doses are evaluated until the trial stops. The trial protocol[#] could specify what might be a maximum number of patients, based on the target range of doses.

Type of subjects

Healthy volunteers are often used, and if safe enough, there could follow another phase I study in patients affected with the disorder of interest. An exception is cancer drug trials, where traditional anti-cancer drugs are first tested in cancer patients because the expected toxic effects make them inappropriate to test in healthy volunteers. Furthermore, healthy people may be able to tolerate cancer drugs at higher doses than a cancer patient, who is already ill. Cancer patients included in phase I studies have usually had

---

[#] A detailed description of the trial design and conduct; see page 160.

A concise guide to clinical trials, First edition. By A. Hackshaw. Published 2009 by Blackwell Publishing, ISBN: 978-1-4051-6774-1.

several previous therapies, but did not respond, so they tend to be less fit than the target group of patients. Therefore, estimates of treatment effectiveness need to be interpreted carefully. Several phase I studies may be conducted, each looking at different aspects of a new therapy. For example, examining the pharmacological effects when the drug is taken with and without food, giving multiple doses, and renal impairment.

Trial subjects must be monitored very closely, and this is usually done by admitting them to a special clinical trials facility, allowing regular examinations over 24 hours or longer, such as blood tests and physical examinations. If there is already evidence on the drug's safety profile, subjects may be seen as outpatients, but they still need to be examined regularly (e.g. at least once a week). Participants are often found through advertisements in the media, and those accepted onto a trial programme are paid for taking part (usually for commercial company trials).

Outcome measures

One or more measures of toxicity are often the common main endpoints. In healthy volunteers a serious adverse event can be any reaction related to the trial drug that requires treatment and the person to be taken off the new drug. This is called a **dose-limiting toxicity (DLT)**. A DLT should occur relatively soon after the drug was administered. In phase I trials based on subjects who are already ill, some adverse events are expected naturally, and so may not be classified as a DLT. The trial protocol should provide clear definitions of toxicity.

The principle aim is to find the **maximum tolerated dose (MTD)**, which can be defined differently. Sometimes, it is the dose at which a pre-specified number of individuals suffer a severe adverse event, indicating that this dose may be too unsafe, so the next lowest dose would be investigated further. This definition can also be called the **maximum administered dose**. At other times, the MTD could be the dose that has an acceptable number of side-effects and is therefore used in further studies. It is useful to be clear about the definition used in a particular trial report.

Many other trial endpoints are measured, including those which monitor drug uptake, metabolism and excretion, for example, body temperature, blood pressure, plasma concentration of the drug and other biological and physiological measurements. There could also be several surrogate markers that provide an initial evaluation of treatment effect, particularly when the study is conducted in patients affected with the disorder of interest. Many variables are examined because the data will be used to determine whether the drug is safe enough and worth investigating further. The timing of the assessments (i.e. how often), especially blood samples, needs to be carefully considered, and is usually fairly frequently early on.

Which doses?

The starting dose for many drug trials is based on animal experiments, and is one that is associated with a specified mortality rate. Different countries

Table 3.1 Fibonacci sequence of numbers and the possible doses for a hypothetical trial.

Fibonacci sequence	Difference between successive numbers	Ratio of successive numbers	Example of a dose (mg) to be used in a phase I trial	Possible modified Fibonacci doses*
1	–	–	3	3
1	0	1	3	3
2	1	2	6	5
3	1	1.5	9	10
5	2	1.667	15	15
8	3	1.600	24	25
13	5	1.625	39	40
21	8	1.615	63	65
34	13	1.619	102	100
55	21	1.618	165	165

*observed Fibonacci dose rounded to the nearest 5 mg.

have different requirements, for example, the US Food and Drug Administration require evidence from at least two mammalian species, including a non-rodent species.[5,6] The starting dose may also be specified in the guidelines. For example, with anti-cancer drugs the initial dose is usually one-tenth of the dose that is associated with 10% of rodents dying in laboratory studies. If a non-rodent species indicates that this dose is too toxic then the starting dose could be one-third or one-sixthof the lowest toxic dose in those species.

There are several methods for determining subsequent doses. One is based on a Fibonacci sequence, a series of numbers found to occur naturally in many biological and ecological systems, for example, the number of petals on flowers. The series starts off with a '0' and '1', then every successive number is the sum of the preceding two numbers. The first 10 numbers in the series are: 0, 1, 1, 2, 3, 5, 8, 13, 21, 34.

While the numbers appear to increase quickly, the relative increase is roughly constant (Table 3.1). After the third dose, each subsequent dose is about two-thirds greater. In practice, the doses are rounded up or down (Table 3.1). This could be referred to as a 'modified Fibonacci' sequence, but the relative increases should still be about two-thirds.

Doses in a trial do not need to follow a Fibonacci sequence. The range could be based on evidence from other studies or previous experience, or they could come from a logrithmic scale (e.g. if the starting dose is 5 mg, subsequent doses could be 10, 20 and 40 mg). The researcher could decide the dose range, and the increase could be greater earlier on. In the example below, the dose increases by about 50% in the three doses after the starting dose of 100 mg, but at higher doses the relative increases are lower:

Dose (mg)	100	150	225	350	450	550
Relative increase	–	50%	50%	55%	29%	22%

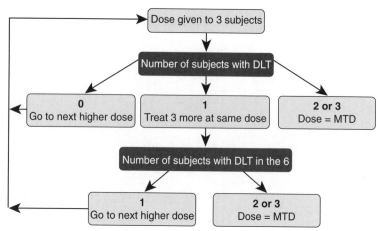

Figure 3.1 Flowchart for a phase I trial using a '3+3' design. MTD (maximum tolerated dose); DLT (dose-limiting toxicity). Doses are increased until the maximum planned dose or MTD is reached.

Conducting the trial

Because the drug has not been previously tested in humans, the protocol needs to be followed carefully to avoid unnecessary harm to the subjects. The subjects who have agreed to participate could also be randomised to the different doses (possibly even a placebo), though subsequent doses should only be given after the current cohort of subjects have been evaluated for safety, after a sufficient time has elapsed. There is a range of designs, from simple to complex. A simple dose-escalation design is a **3 + 3 design**.

The '3+3' dose escalation scheme is a classical approach. It is based on observing how many subjects in each group have a DLT before deciding whether to keep the current dose or move to a higher dose. It is called '3+3' because subjects are recruited in groups of three or six, as shown in Figure 3.1.

In this design, the decision rules to stop or continue to a higher dose are based on a conventional toxicity risk of 1 in 3. If a different risk were assumed, such as 1 in 4, the decision rules would need to change. While this design is simple, there are limitations. If the starting dose is too low, there may be no DLTs until after several doses have been administered. Therefore several subjects would have been treated without providing much information about the MTD of the new drug, and the trial would take longer. There also is a chance that the true MTD could be higher than the one indicated in a particular trial, i.e. the study stops too early. If the drug is not too toxic, the design can be adapted to reduce the probability of stopping early.

There are several other variations on these designs,[3] e.g. accelerated titration, but whichever is used, the safety stopping rules should be clearly specified before the trial begins, to minimise the possibility of researcher bias towards higher (and possibly more unsafe) doses. While these types of

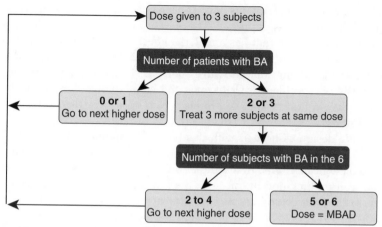

Figure 3.2 Flowchart for a phase I trial based on examining a biological endpoint. MBAD (minimum biologically active dose); BA (biological activity). Doses are increased until the maximum planned dose or MBAD is reached.

designs are simple to use and easy to interpret, they have been criticised for being inefficient. Sometimes the starting and subsequent early doses are too low, so many subjects are treated before any activity (safety or efficacy) is observed.

There are more complex dose-escalation designs that are believed to be more efficient. These include the **continuous reassessment method** and those based on Bayesian methods. They are based on statistical modelling and assume a mathematical relationship between dose and the chance of having a DLT at each dose; often a sigmoid (flattened S-shaped) curve. At early doses, a lack of toxicities indicates that subsequent doses could be made greater than those based on, say, a Fibonacci sequence. After each cohort of subjects has been evaluated, the actual shape of the dose-response curve is re-estimated, in order to reach the MTD quicker. Sometimes, there may only be one subject per dose, so that fewer patients are needed than the simpler designs. However, a limitation of these methods is that it may be difficult to get enough information about the pharmacological actions of the drug with only one subject per dose.[4]

Once the MTD has been determined, it might be useful to test the dose on a further group of, say, 10 subjects, to obtain a clearer view of the safety profile before proceeding to a larger study and perhaps also an examination of efficacy.

3.2 Non-toxicity endpoints

The above designs are used to identify the maximum tolerated dose when using drugs or exposures with expected toxicities. As new safer therapies are developed, biological endpoints or pharmacological measures, i.e. markers of drug activity, may be as important. The objective of the trial could then be to find the *minimum* dose that has a material effect on the biological endpoint. This is sometimes called the **minimum biologically active dose (MBAD)**. Rather than identifying subjects who exhibit a DLT, an endpoint of **biological activity (BA)** is specified. Toxicity must still be monitored closely, but there may be other indicators that determine which dose is carried forward to a phase II study.

A simple design associated with this type of endpoint is the '5/6 design' (Figure 3.3).[3] The MBAD is chosen when five out of six subjects exhibit a pre-defined biological activity. An example could be changes in Ki67, a marker of tumour cell proliferation in cancer. If the Ki67 for a patient decreases from, say, 50 to 25%, this could indicate biological activity of a new treatment.

3.3 Statistical analysis and reporting the trial results

There should be a summary of the characteristics of the subjects, details of the side-effects observed (including severity), and a description of the following pharmacological effects:

- Pharmacodynamics: physical or biological measures that show the effect of the new drug on the body (this could include efficacy)
- Pharmacokinetics: physical or biological measures that show how the body deals with the new drug.

Pharmacokinetics can be presented as a plasma concentration–time curve, which plots blood levels of the new drug against time since administration, showing how much of the drug gets into the blood and what happens to these levels over time (Figure 3.3). The following measures can be obtained from this type of curve, for each subject:[2]

- area under the curve (AUC), indicating total drug exposure
- Cmax, the highest concentration level
- Tmax, the time at which Cmax occurs

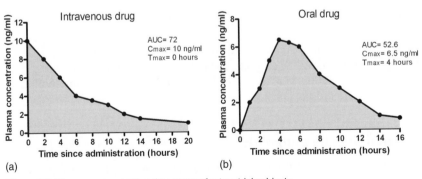

(a)   (b)

Figure 3.3 Plasma concentration-time curves for two trial subjects.

- terminal half-life ($t_{1/2}$), the time it takes for the plasma concentration to decrease by 50% in the final part of the curve, when the drug is being eliminated (here, the curve may appear as a straight line if using a log transformation of the plasma levels).

Other measures are clearance (CL), the rate at which the drug is removed from the plasma as it is metabolised or excreted ($CL = dose/AUC$); volume of distribution (V), the amount of drug in the body divided by the plasma concentration; and bioavailability (F), the percentage of administered dose that gets into the systemic circulation (e.g. an intravenous drug should have $F = 100\%$).[2]

Summary curves and statistics can be produced across all subjects (e.g. the mean AUC). Showing that AUC increases proportionally with dose (i.e. AUC doubles as the dose doubles), makes it easier to describe and model the effect of the drug, and plan further early phase studies. There could also be a description of how the body metabolises the drug (i.e. what molecules the drug changes to), and the process and speed of excretion.

Table 3.2 Example of a phase I trial.[7]

Study feature	Example
Target disease	Parkinson's disease
Drug being investigated	BAY 63-9044, a new $5\text{-}HT_{1a}$-receptor agonist (has neuroprotective and symptomatic effects)
Aim	To determine the maximum tolerated dose
Design	First-in-man trial of male healthy volunteers, aged 18–45 years (randomised study)
Treatment doses investigated	0.25, 0.50, 1.20, 2.50, 5.00 mg and placebo
Definition of dose-limiting toxicity, DLT (i.e. treatment-related side-effects)	Any drug-related adverse event (graded mild, moderate, severe)
Number of subjects	$N = 45$
Main result	There were no serious adverse events
	The number of mild or moderate events out of the number of subjects in the cohort were: Placebo $n = 0/14$ 0.25 mg $n = 2/7$ 0.50 $n = 0/7$ 1.20 $n = 0/6$ 2.50 $n = 1/5$ 5.00 $n = 5/6$
Conclusion	There were too many subjects with adverse events in the 5 mg dose group.
	A dose of 2.5 mg should be used in further studies.

An example of a phase I trial is given in Table 3.2.[7] Five out of six patients suffered an adverse event at the highest dose of 5 mg, therefore the next lowest dose (2.5 mg) would be recommended for further investigation.

3.4 Summary points

• Phase I studies are small and aim to provide a first assessment of safety in human subjects
• There are simple designs for determining the dose of a new drug that has an acceptable number of serious side-effects
• Trials of new, safer therapies may need to have different biological endpoints as well as toxicity
• Reports of phase I studies should provide clear information on the pharmacological properties of a new drug, including plasma concentration curves over time, and details of adverse events.

References

1. O'Grady J, Joubert PH (Eds). *Handbook of Phase 1 and 2 Clinical Drug Trials*. CRC Press Inc., 1997.
2. Griffin JP, O'Grady J (Eds). *The textbook of pharmaceutical medicine*. BMJ Books, Blackwell Publishing, 5th edn, 2006.
3. Eisenhauer EA, Twelves C, Buyse M. *Phase I cancer clinical trials: a practical guide*. Oxford University Press, 2006.
4. Eisenhauer EA, O'Dwyer PJ, Christian M, Humphrey JS. Phase I clinical trial design in cancer drug development. *J Clin Oncol* 2000; **18**:684–692.
5. www.fda.gov/cder/guidance/pt1.pdf
6. http://www.fda.gov/cder/guidance/7086fnl.pdf
7. Wensing G, Haase C, Brendel E, Bottcher MF. Pupillography as a sensitive, non-invasive biomarker in healthy volunteers: first-in-man study of BAY 63-9044, a new 5-HT$_{1a}$-receptor agonist with dopamine agnostic properties. *Eur J Clin Pharmacol* 2007; **63**:1123–1128.

CHAPTER 4

Design and analysis of phase II trials

Phase II trials are useful in examining the potential effectiveness of an intervention before embarking on a large, expensive phase III trial. They are common in oncology, and many of the designs and statistical issues have been based on cancer studies.

4.1 Purpose of phase II studies

The aim is to obtain *preliminary* evidence on whether a new treatment might be effective, i.e. whether it can influence a clinically important outcome measure, such as mortality, or reduce the severity of a disease. Safety should still be monitored closely. The results of a phase II study often help design a phase III trial.

Phase II studies may also be **pilot** (or **feasibility**) **studies**, used to assess whether a phase III trial is likely to be successful. The study is designed and conducted in a similar manner to a phase III trial (Chapter 5), but the protocol specifies that an early assessment is made after a proportion of subjects have been recruited first (e.g. 25%), or the trial has run for a fixed length of time. A formal sample size calculation for this part of the study is not normally necessary.

Pilot studies often raise issues that require investigation, for example, examining the proportion of eligible subjects approached who agree to participate (i.e. the **acceptance** or **uptake rate**), and if accrual is low, what might be the likely reasons for this. Consider a phase III trial requiring 600 subjects to be recruited over four years. The pilot phase could be conducted to see whether a recruitment rate of 15 subjects per month is likely. The endpoint is 'monthly accrual rate' assessed, say, 12 months after recruitment started, ignoring the expected low initial accrual rates during trial set up (say 60 in the first year). If the uptake rate is low, ways could be found to encourage participation, perhaps by changing the wording of the patient information sheet (see page 161). In the remainder of this chapter only phase II studies examining efficacy and safety are discussed.

4.2 Design

There are several phase II designs, and a discussion is found in various sources (though some are aimed at statisticians).[1–8] Most methods are intended for

A concise guide to clinical trials, First edition. By A. Hackshaw. Published 2009 by Blackwell Publishing, ISBN: 978-1-4051-6774-1.

Box 4.1 Example of a two-stage phase II design

The response rate for a new treatment should not be lower than 20%, the rate associated with standard therapy. The new intervention should have a response rate of at least 35%. Using these estimates, 5% level of statistical significance and 80% power (page 43) produces the following design:

Stage 1 :   Recruit and treat 22 subjects
　　　　　　If ≥6 respond, continue trial to Stage 2 (treatment might be effective enough)
　　　　　　If ≤5 respond, stop trial early (treatment unlikely to be effective enough)

Stage 2 :   Recruit a further 50 patients, to make 72 in total
　　　　　　If ≥20 respond consider further investigation

The method is described in reference 11.

---

studies examining whether a new intervention is likely to be better than current treatments, based on an improvement in disease status, or fewer side-effects.

Single-arm study

The simplest design has only one arm: all subjects are given the new intervention. The advantage is that all resources, i.e. subjects and financial costs, are concentrated on one group. Some designs also specify how many subjects should respond to the new treatment in order to justify further investigation. For example, if a new intervention has an expected treatment response rate of 35% and the percentage of subjects who currently respond is 20%, the sample size would be 56 subjects, of which ≥17 need to respond to indicate that the **true** response rate is greater than 20%.[#] If, however, there are only five responders it is unlikely that the treatment is effective. (The definition of 'response' will depend on the trial endpoint used.)

Single-arm two-stage study

Although single-arm phase II studies usually have about 30–70 subjects, it may be preferable to stop the trial early. In a two-stage design, the intervention is first tested on a small number of subjects, and the subjects are assessed at the end of this stage (Box 4.1). If a certain number respond, the trial continues and a second group of subjects is recruited, otherwise the trial stops: this is

---

[#] 17 out of 56 is 30%, but the calculated one-sided 95% confidence interval (discussed later in this chapter), has a lower limit of 20.4%. The lower limit excludes the possibility of a true underlying rate of 20% with sufficient certainty – i.e. the new treatment response rate is likely to be greater than 20%.

referred to as a **stopping rule**. This design is used when the outcome is based on 'counting people' (i.e. binary data). Two-stage designs are useful when the new intervention might have serious side-effects or is expensive, because only a few subjects are given such a therapy, which may have no true benefit. A practical limitation is that after the first stage is reached, centres probably need to stop recruiting further patients until the initial assessment is made. They then need to re-start recruiting if enough subjects respond. There are logistical issues associated with temporarily halting a study.

However, the decision to continue to Stage 2 may hinge on the response of only one or two subjects. In Box 4.1, suppose there are five responders during Stage 1, but there really is a beneficial effect of the treatment. If the stopping rule is strictly adhered to, an effective treatment would not be studied further and future patients would not benefit. The alternative is also possible. A truly ineffective treatment is investigated further because a sufficient number of subjects happened to show a response in Stage 1, though this is probably of less importance.

Randomised phase II trial with control arm

There are two trial groups; the new intervention and a control (standard treatment or placebo). The control arm is often used when it is not well known how subjects respond generally. The results found in each arm are used to design the corresponding arms in a phase III trial, in particular determining sample size (see Chapter 5). By randomising subjects to the trial arms, some comparison could be made at the end of the study, although this will not determine whether the new intervention is better. This design also provides information on recruitment rates, subjects' willingness to participate in a randomised study, and possible logistical problems, all of which could help future studies.

Randomised phase II trial with several intervention arms

Two or more new treatments could be examined simultaneously. Each arm is designed as a single-arm study, and subjects are randomised to the different groups, with the same advantages as above. One or more of the new treatments are identified that could be investigated further. This design is sometimes called 'pick the winner', though there is not necessarily a single 'winner'. The primary intention is not to directly compare the results between the new treatment arms. Deciding which treatment should be taken further is determined in the same way as with a single-arm phase II study, i.e. whether the treatment response rate in each arm exceeds the expected response associated with standard treatments. This design could also include a control arm using standard treatment or placebo.

Randomised phase II trial with several intervention arms: two-stage design

This is an extension of the single-arm two-stage design. At the first stage, a few subjects (specified by the sample size calculation) are randomised to each of the new treatments. An assessment of efficacy is made, and those treatments that seem effective enough proceed to Stage 2, though not all will past the first stage (another form of 'pick the winner').

Types of phase II trials

- Single arm
- Single arm, two-stage design
- Randomised phase II with control arm
- Randomised phase II with several new treatment arms*
- Randomised phase II with several new treatment arms, two-stage design.*

*could include a control arm (standard treatment or placebo)

4.3 Choosing outcome measures

Phase II studies should be conducted in a relatively short space of time, and the main endpoint should be compatible with this, as well as being clinically relevant. Therefore, several surrogate endpoints can be used (page 17). Observed changes in a validated surrogate endpoint may indicate an effect on a true endpoint. Similarly, if a new treatment appears to have no effect on a surrogate marker, it is unlikely that it would have an effect on a true endpoint. There may be several endpoints because the aim is to have a preliminary evaluation of the new intervention, and sufficient information is needed to decide whether a larger phase III trial is justified.

4.4 Sample size

There are various methods for estimating how many subjects should be recruited. This depends on the study design employed (single or two-stage), and the type of outcome measure. Two treatment effects are specified (i.e. two proportions or two mean values):

- One that is thought to be associated with the new intervention. This may come from prior evidence, or it may be the minimum effect that would be considered clinically important
- One that is considered to be the lowest acceptable level, usually the same as that for current treatments or standard of care. The new treatment needs to be more effective than this. The sample size method assumes that this effect is known with certainty.

A fundamental difference between randomised phase II and III trials is that the sample-size calculation for phase III studies *assumes* that the treatment effect in each arm is not known with certainty, even though there is some knowledge of this in the standard treatment group (see page 10). In phase II studies, the sample-size calculation assumes there is only one area of uncertainty, i.e. the new intervention arm. This is why the sample size is always larger in a phase III trial: the treatment effect in *each* trial arm will have some imprecision when trying to estimate the true effects.

Information is required on two other factors:

Statistical significance level. This is often set at 5%. If a new treatment is believed to have a response rate of 35%, but it really has a response rate which is no greater than the standard treatment (e.g. 20% response rate), there would be a 5% probability of finding a difference as large as 15 percentage points just by chance.[#] (This is called a Type I error.) It is assumed that a mistake would be made by concluding that the new intervention is better than standard treatments, when in fact it is not, so a **one-sided** significance level is used. In many phase III trials, a **two-sided** significance level is used, because a mistake is made by concluding that the new intervention is better or worse than the control group, when there really is no difference between them (see Chapter 5).

Power. This is the chance of finding an effect in the study if a true effect really exists. This is set at a high level, 80 or 90%. (The converse, 20 or 10% is called a Type II error, the chance of missing an effect if it exists.) In the example above, there could be an 80% chance of finding a difference ≥ 15 percentage points, if the true response rate is 35%.

Power

At the end of the trial we want to say:

'A comparison of the observed response rate of 35% (new intervention) compared with the known[*] response of 20% (control) is statistically significant at the 5% level.'

$$\downarrow$$

We want an 80% probability of being able to make this statement (80% power) if there really is a difference of this magnitude.

[*]assumed to be known with certainty

There are various statistical formulae to calculate sample size[7–11], some of which come with free software[7], and commercially software is available.[12–13]

Calculating the sample size

When the outcome measure involves counting people, the specified percentage (or proportion) associated with the new treatment and standard therapy

---

[#]'15 percentage points' is a better way of describing the effect than '15%' when comparing two percentages. It avoids the possible confusion over whether the rate for the new treatment is 20% + 15% = 35%, rather than 15% greater than 20%, which would be 20% × 1.15 = 23%.

Table 4.1 Sample sizes for a phase II study, where the endpoint is based on 'counting people'. The table shows the number of subjects that need to be given the new treatment (based on a 5% one-sided level of statistical significance), from A'Hern.[9]

		80% power	90% power
Counting people			
% standard treatment (assumed to be known)	% expected in new intervention		
10	20	78 (13)	109 (17)
	25	40 (8)	55 (10)
	30	25 (6)	33 (7)
30	40	141 (52)	193 (69)
	45	67 (27)	93 (36)
	50	39 (17)	53 (22)
50	60	158 (90)	213 (119)
	65	69 (42)	93 (55)
	70	37 (24)	53 (33)

If a randomised phase II trial with a control arm is used, the total study size is usually double the number of subjects in the above table.

The numbers in brackets are the number of observed responses needed at the end of the trial to help justify further investigation of the new treatment (it ensures that the lower limit of a one-sided confidence interval exceeds the response rate in the standard treatment arm). Another method is by Fleming[10], though both approaches give similar sample sizes as they get larger.

are used in the sample-size calculation. Examples are shown in Table 4.1. When taking measurements on people, the specified means and the standard deviation are required, which are converted into a **standardised difference**.

Standardised difference
$$= \frac{(\text{expected mean in intervention group}) - (\text{known mean using standard treatment})}{\text{standard deviation of the measurement}}$$

For example, suppose a new diet aims to reduce body weight to 83 kg. If the usual average weight is 85 kg, with standard deviation of 5 kg, the standardised difference is $(83 - 85)/5 = -0.4$. The simplest sample size method assumes that the endpoint has a Normal distribution. If it clearly does not, then non-parametric methods should be used, which are more complex.

Sample size based on 'taking measurements on people' endpoints could be calculated using a one-sample t-test. For example, the number of subjects that need to be given a new therapy are 101, 40 and 27 for standardised differences of 0.25, 0.40 and 0.50 respectively (80% power and one-sided 5% level).

When estimating sample size for a 'time-to-event' endpoint, a simple approach is to use the 'counting people' category, allowing the use of standard methods. Consider a new therapy for Alzheimer's disease, where the trial endpoint is time to progression. The percentage of patients who have progressed (or not progressed) at a certain time point, say six months, is used though all patients need to be followed for six months.

If the median times are known, they can be converted to an event rate at a specific time point. Suppose the expected median time to progression using the new treatment is eight months, but the six-month progression-free rate is required, then:

- Progression-free rate at y months = exponential $[(\log_e 0.5 \times y)/\text{median progression}]$[#]
- Progression-free rate at six months = exponential $[(\log_e 0.5 \times 6)/8] = 0.59$ or 59%

  (the progression rate at six months = $100 - 59\% = 41\%$).

If the median using standard therapy is five months (assumed to be known with certainty), the six-month progression-free rate is 44%.

The sample size can be estimated using 59 vs 44% (about 70 patients).[9]

Table 4.2 shows examples of sample size descriptions for different trial designs. In the last example, the researcher chooses the number of patients in the control arm, and it often just happens to be the same as the intervention arm. There is no scientific justification for this. They are made the same because this makes it easier to describe and conduct the trial, particularly if a placebo group is used, and the trial will look more similar to the possible subsequent phase III trial. The ratio of subjects in the new intervention and control arm could be 2:1. In phase III trials the number of subjects in both arms come from the statistical method used to estimate sample size.

Information needed to calculate sample size

- Expected effect in the new intervention group
- The effect in patients given standard treatments (assumed to be known with certainty)
- Significance level (usually 5%, at the one-sided level)
- Power (usually 80% or 90%).

Sample-size estimation is not an exact science. It is dependent on the input parameters, for example, the estimated effect in the test arm, and the known effect using standard treatment. If either of these is far from the true values, the sample size will be too small or too large. Few trials produce effects that

---

[#]Assumes that progression (or any other time-to-event measure) has an exponential distribution.

Table 4.2 Hypothetical examples of sample size descriptions that can be used in a grant application or trial protocol.

Type of phase II study *Outcome measure category* *Trial endpoint*	*Description* (the numbers in bold are those needed for the sample size calculation, using formulae or software, to produce the number of subjects required, and sometimes the number of required treatment responders)
Single arm Counting people Progression rate (%)	The percentage of Alzheimer's patients who are expected to progress after one year with a new Drug A is **15%**. The percentage who usually progress is **25%.** Drug A should not have a progression rate as high as this. A single-arm study would require 103 patients to show a decrease from 25 to 15% as statistically significant at the **5%** level (**one-sided**) with **80%** power. If at most 15 patients progress, then a larger trial might be justified.[#]
Single arm Taking measurements on people Body weight (kg)	Diet B is expected to reduce body weight by 2 kg in women aged 20–40 years. Body weight is Normally distributed and the mean weight in women is generally about 70 kg, with a standard deviation of 5 kg. The aim is to reduce body weight to 68 kg. A single-arm study would require 40 subjects to show a **standardised difference of 0.4** [(68–70-)/5], with **80%** power and a **one-sided 5%** level of statistical significance.
Single arm two-stage Counting people Tumour response rate (%)	The percentage of patients with an advanced sub-type of ovarian cancer who are expected to have a partial/complete tumour response after standard treatment is about 20%. A new Therapy F is expected to increase this to 35%. Using a two-stage design with (**80%** power and **one-sided 5%** significance level) the following design is employed. 22 patients are recruited in Stage 1. If 6 or more patients respond, then a further 50 patients are recruited (Stage 2), to make 72 in total. If 20 or more respond out of 72 then a larger trial would be worthwhile.
Randomised phase II with control arm Counting people Progression-free survival rate (%)	The percentage of patients with pancreatic cancer who are alive and progression-free is normally 20% after 1 year. Therapy G is expected to increase this to 35%. Fifty-six patients need to be given Therapy G in a phase II study with **80%** power and **one-sided** test of statistical significance at the **5%** level. If at least 17 patients remain alive and progression-free, then a larger trial might be justified.

Because this type of cancer is relatively uncommon, the progression-free survival rate using standard treatments is not known with sufficient reliability. A control arm that has the same number of patients as the new treatment arm, i.e. 56 patients, will be used. Therefore, the trial will have 112 patients in total. To allow an unbiased comparison at the end of the study, patients will be randomised to both arms, acknowledging that the study is not powered for such a comparison. |

[#]Sample size methods for 'counting people' endpoints are often based on those that are 'positive' (e.g. respond to treatment or are alive). In this example, the endpoint is 'negative', so 85% and 75% are used in the calculation, instead of 15 and 25%.

It is worthwhile providing references to the effect using standard treatments from the literature or unpublished work, where possible.

are identical to the sample-size parameters. Therefore, given the natural variability in how subjects respond to treatments, it should not matter whether the estimated sample size is 50 or 55, but rather whether it is 50 or 100. Also, the results should be interpreted in the context of the type of patients that were entered into the study since they might, for example, have a lower response rate than that used in the sample-size calculation because they had a poorer prognosis than originally anticipated.

4.5 Stopping early for toxicity

When testing a new drug or medical device, a **stopping rule** for toxicity could be incorporated. The trial stops early if the number of subjects who suffer a severe treatment-related adverse event exceeds a pre-specified level. The rule can be estimated using the sample size for efficacy. Suppose the sample size is 56 patients (to compare a response rate of 35% with 20%, new vs control treatments respectively). It is then necessary to specify what is considered to be an unacceptable toxicity rate – for example, more than 30% – and use a calculation based on the 'binomial distribution'. This gives the probability of seeing 'x' or more people with an adverse event, by chance, *assuming* that the underlying (true) toxicity rate is 'p' (e.g. 30%). In the example, the probabilities of seeing at least 20 people with an adverse event, out of 56, are as follows:

Number of subjects with an adverse event	20	21	22	23	24	25
Probability of seeing this number or greater	0.21	0.14	0.09	0.051	0.028	0.01

Observing 20 or 21 affected subjects is consistent with a true rate of 30% because this could occur by chance. The trial would not stop early. However, as soon as 24 or 25 patients have an event, this is evidence that the true rate is probably greater than 30%. For example, the likelihood of seeing ≥ 24 events by chance, among 56 patients, is 0.028 *if the underlying rate were 30%*. Because this is a small probability (less than 5%[#]), it can be concluded that the true rate is likely to exceed 30%. Consideration should then be given to stopping early.

4.6 Statistical analysis

A description of the subject population should be provided, usually as a table summarising baseline characteristics, such as the age and gender distribution and other factors relevant to the disease of interest (for example, disease stage). The following focuses on how to analyse and interpret the results for a single trial arm. Statistical analyses for comparing two arms are discussed in Chapter 7.

The data is often analysed on an **intention-to-treat** basis, i.e. trial subjects are included in the analysis whether or not they actually took the new

---

[#]5% is the accepted cut-off; see also statistical significance on page 112.

treatment. It may also be useful to look at efficacy and toxicity in subjects who did take the trial treatment (a **per-protocol analysis**). Both approaches are discussed on page 116.

In research, '**population**' refers to the set of all people of interest, and to whom a new intervention could be given. When conducting a trial, a **sample** of subjects is taken from the **population**. Data from the sample is used to make inferences, not just about the individuals in the sample, but about the whole population of interest. For example, in examining a new drug to alleviate pain in adults with arthritis, a sample of patients is selected for the trial, but the aim is to determine the effect of the drug in all patients, now and in the future. It is not possible to study every adult with arthritis, so there will always be some uncertainty in what can be inferred about the population from the sample in the trial:

- Would the same result emerge in another group of subjects given the new intervention?
- Can the *true* treatment effect be estimated?

Natural variation between people and how they respond to the same treatment matters a great deal when interpreting research data (see page 4). Two statistical parameters, called **standard error** and the **confidence interval**, allow this variability to be taken into account.

Analysing outcome measures based on counting people

The summary statistic is a simple percentage or proportion. In a group of 50 subjects given the new intervention, if 28 responded (however defined), the observed response rate is 56% (28/50). An estimate of the **true** or **population** proportion is needed. The true value is unlikely to be 56% exactly, but it is hoped that it would be close.

The standard error of the true proportion quantifies how far the observed value is expected to be from the true value, given the results of the trial with a certain sample size. (This is done using assumptions about the data and established mathematical properties.) A standard error is used to produce a **confidence interval (CI)**. A trial based on every relevant subject ever would yield the true proportion. There would be no uncertainty and the standard error would be zero.

What are the implications of conducting a trial on a sample of people?

A **CI for the true proportion** is a range within which the true proportion is expected to lie:

95% CI = observed proportion $\pm$ 1.96 $\times$ standard error

If the response rate is 56% (28/50), the **95% CI** is 42% to 70% (see page 205 for the calculation). From this particular trial, the best estimate of the true proportion of responders is 56%, but there is 95% certainty that the true value

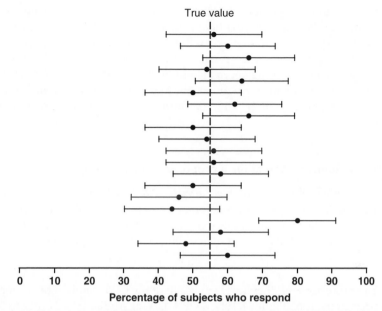

Figure 4.1 The percentage of subjects who respond to a new treatment in 20 hypothetical phase II trials, each based on 50 subjects. Each dot represents the observed percentage, and the ends of the line are the lower and upper limits of the 95% confidence interval (two-sided). It is assumed that the true effect of the new treatment is known to be 55%, indicated by the vertical dashed line.

lies somewhere between 42 and 70%.[#] This also means that the range could get the wrong answer 5% of the time. A conservative estimate is that 42% of all subjects are expected to respond, but as many as 70% could respond.

This is a **two-sided** CI, and one that is commonly reported. The new intervention could be better or worse than the standard therapy. In phase II studies the main interest is in whether the new intervention is likely to be better, so researchers may also examine a **one-sided** CI. For this, only the upper or lower limit is needed, depending on which direction indicates benefit in relation to standard therapy. In the example, the objective is for the proportion responding to be greater than that using the standard treatment, so the lower limit is required. It is 44%, which should be higher than the response rate for standard treatments to justify further investigation.

Figure 4.1 illustrates the concept of confidence intervals using the one given above (shown at the top of the diagram) and 19 hypothetical studies. For illustrative purposes, the true response rate is assumed to be known: 55%. Each of the 20 trials is trying to estimate this. Some will have an estimate above 55%,

---

[#]The strict definition is that 95% of such intervals will contain the true proportion, but it is often easier to interpret confidence intervals using the definition in the main text; little is lost by this.

others below, and occasionally 55% exactly, but all have CIs that include 55%, except one trial (fourth from the bottom). Because 95% CIs are used, 5% of them (1 in every 20) are expected to exclude the true effect, just by chance.

A 95% CI is commonly used because a 5% error rate is considered sufficiently low. There is nothing special about '95%'; sometimes 90% or 99% CIs are used. For moderate to large studies, the multiplier '1.96' is associated with using a two-sided 95% range. Different multipliers are needed for different levels of confidence.

95% Confidence interval for a proportion or percentage

A range of plausible values for the **true** value based on the observed data. It is a range within which the true proportion is expected to lie with a high degree of certainty. If confidence intervals were calculated from many different studies of the same size, 95% of them should contain the true proportion.

The standard error and, therefore, the width of the CI depend on the number of subjects in the trial. Figure 4.2 shows 95% CIs for studies based on 10 to 500

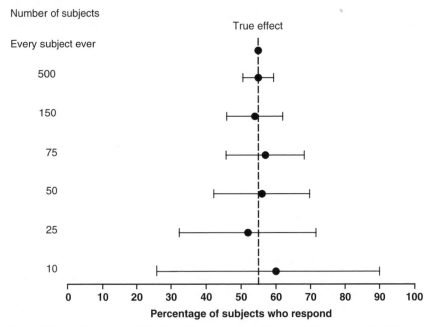

Figure 4.2 Counting people: Estimates of the proportion who respond to a new treatment in hypothetical phase II trials of different sizes. Each dot represents the estimate of the treatment effect, and the ends of the line are the lower and upper limits of the 95% confidence interval (two-sided). It is assumed that the true effect of the new treatment is known to be 55%, indicated by the vertical dashed line.

subjects. If the true effect were known there would be no confidence interval. The larger the study, the greater the confidence that the observed estimate is closer to the true value, so the range becomes narrower. A trial with few subjects produces a wide CI, which reflects the lack of sufficient certainty over the true value. Conclusions based on wide CIs (e.g. 95% CI 5% to 60%) are difficult to interpret because the possible true proportion could be very low or high. Such small studies can justly be described as uninformative because they do not provide reliable information on the likely true value.

Large study ⟶ small standard error ⟶ narrow confidence interval
Small study ⟶ large standard error ⟶ wide confidence interval

---

Once the 95% CI is estimated, it is examined to see if it contains the response rate for standard treatment. An example is given in Box 4.2. When there are two or more new treatments, each 95% CI is examined to observe which exclude and which include the expected effect for the standard treatment.

Box 4.2 Example of a phase II trial[14]

Objective: To examine the effect of using thalidomide in treating small cell lung cancer, when added to standard chemotherapy

Trial design: Single-arm phase II study

Outcome measure: Tumour response rate (complete or partial remission)

Sample size: Thalidomide should have a response rate greater than 45% (standard treatments). A value as large as 70% would indicate that it would be worthwhile investigating further in a large phase III trial. A sample size of 24 patients is required to detect this difference (with 80% power and 5% level of statistical significance, one-sided test).

Results: 25 patients were recruited of whom 17 had a tumour response
Response rate = 68% (17/25)
One-sided 95% confidence interval (CI): lower limit is 50%
Two-sided 95% CI = 46 to 85%

Interpretation: The observed response rate was high (68%). The one-sided lower limit is 50%, which means that enough patients had a tumour response (17) to suggest that thalidomide could be associated with a true rate that is greater than 45%. The observed rate is also close to the target rate of 70%. The two-sided CI indicates that the true rate could be as high as 85%.

Recommendation: Thalidomide is worth further investigation

(95% CIs were calculated using an exact method)

Sometimes a greater level of confidence is used, such as a 97.5%, to partly allow for having multiple comparisons, which increases the chance of finding an effect, when there really is none. In deciding which merit further study, the one(s) with the largest observed effect might be selected. If they all appear to be better than the standard treatment, the side-effects of each treatment, and the feasibility of conducting a larger trial with several groups, may be considered in choosing which to take forward.

Analysing outcome measures based on taking measurements on people

When the endpoint involves taking measurements on people, the data can be summarised by the **mean** and **standard deviation** (Chapter 2). In the same way that a single proportion observed in a trial will be an estimate of the true proportion, an observed mean value from a trial will be an estimate of the **true mean**. The **standard error** of the mean quantifies how far the observed mean is expected to be from the true value, and is used to estimate a CI for the true mean:

95% CI = observed mean $\pm$ 1.96 $\times$ standard error

What are the implications of conducting a trial on a sample of patients?

Suppose a new pain killer in adults with chronic back pain is evaluated using a phase II study of 40 patients, and the endpoint is pain score (using a visual analogue scale, 0 to 100 mm; 0 represents no pain and 100 is maximum pain). At the end of the trial the observed mean pain score is 34 mm, with a standard deviation of 18 mm (see page 205 for calculation).

Using the results from this particular study, the true mean VAS score associated with the new drug could be 34 mm, but whatever it is, there is 95% certainty that the true value is somewhere between 28 and 40 mm. For a one-sided CI the VAS score should be lower than with standard treatment, so the upper limit is required: 39 mm (34 + 1.645 $\times$ 2.8). If the mean VAS associated with standard treatment is 50 mm, the trial results indicate that the new treatment could be better, because the value is lower.

If there were 20 phase II trials examining the new pain killer, each based on 40 patients, they would look similar to those in Figure 4.1, in that 19 would contain the true mean value. But by chance, 1 in 20 studies (5%) could get the wrong answer; i.e. it will miss the true mean value.

Standard deviation and standard error are sometimes confused, but they have very different meanings:
- Standard deviation indicates how much the data is naturally spread out about the mean value (i.e. natural variability between people)
- Standard error relates not to the spread of the data, but to the accuracy with which it is possible to estimate the true mean, given a trial of a certain sample size.

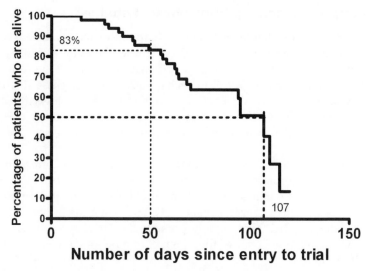

Figure 4.3 Kaplan–Meier plot of the survival times for 50 patients (each death is shown by a vertical drop).

Analysing outcome measures based on time-to-event data

When the endpoint involves measuring the time until an event occurs, a Kaplan–Meier plot, median survival or survival rate at a specific time point are used.[#] Figure 4.3 shows the survival curve for 50 subjects. The median survival is 107 days, and the 95% CI is 70 to 115 days (calculated using statistical software, because the formula is not simple). Using the results from this particular trial, the true median is estimated as 107 days, but there is 95% certainty that the true value is somewhere between 70 and 115 days.

The median time is useful when there are many events, and they occur continuously throughout the follow-up period, such as in studies of patients with advanced disease. Otherwise, it can be skewed by only one or two events, and therefore be unreliable.

The survival rate at 50 days is 83%, and the 95% CI for the true survival rate is 72 to 94%. It should be noted that a rate only applies to a single time point, so could be affected by chance variation. When the median survival is not reached, or it is too dependent on one or two events, the survival rate at a critical time point is more appropriate. The specified time point should be one that is clinically relevant and chosen before the trial starts. The event rate (here, death rate) could also be reported. It is 100 minus the survival rate: 17%, 95% CI: 6 to 28%.

[#]The word 'survival' used here refers to any event of interest occurring, not just death (see page 27).

4.7 Interpreting and reporting phase II studies

Phase II trial reports should include a description of the characteristics of the trial subjects, and summary tables on efficacy and side-effects. Confidence intervals should be reported for the main endpoints. The results of a phase II trial are used to *guide* researchers on whether a phase III trial is needed, which will eventually confirm or refute the early evidence that the new treatment might be effective. A phase II study can also help to design a subsequent larger trial, in terms of outcome measures, sample size and trial conduct.

Many phase II studies are conducted in a few specialist centres, and by experienced health professionals. Therefore, an observed beneficial treatment effect, especially if the trial is not blind, may not be found in routine practice, or the size of the effect is over-estimated. Natural variation in how patients respond to the same treatment, and the possible effect of bias, mean that phase II data, which are based on a relatively small number of patients, should be interpreted carefully.

When the outcome measure involves counting people, the statistical methods used to estimate sample size can also indicate how many events need to be observed to justify further studies. From Table 4.1, 78 subjects are required if the expected response of the new treatment is 20%, and the response using standard therapy is 10%. Seeing at least 13 responders should provide sufficient evidence to warrant further investigation. However, if 12 or even 11 respond, further study should not automatically be ruled out, particularly if the subjects had a poorer prognosis than originally anticipated. Similarly, 13 or 14 responders may not necessarily lead to further studies. The decision to proceed to a phase III trial should be based on other endpoints, such as side-effects, recruitment and patient acceptability, in addition to the response rate.

When phase II trials involve randomising patients to the new and standard treatments, researchers almost always directly compare the outcome measure between the trial groups, and report effect sizes and p-values (see Chapter 7). Although this can be informative, there is sometimes a temptation to conclude that the new treatment is effective. Phase II studies are not designed to provide this kind of definitive evidence. The results could be a chance finding or, more likely, the treatment effect is over-estimated. Care should be taken not to report a randomised phase II study that shows a statistically significant effect as if it were a confirmatory phase III trial, and make undue claims about efficacy. This could prevent further study, and some health professionals may wrongly choose to change practice on the basis of insufficient evidence, and consider conducting a larger phase III study unethical. However, because the number of subjects in the study is relatively small, other professionals will remain unconvinced, and the clinical community as a whole could be left in a state of uncertainty – an unsatisfactory position.

Box 4.3 Example of comparing evidence from phase II and III trials[14,15]

Thalidomide and advanced small cell lung cancer

Two small single-arm phase II trials and a small randomised placebo-controlled trial consistently suggested that thalidomide could greatly increase survival time when used with standard chemotherapy; patients were living noticeably longer than expected.

The percentages of patients surviving to one year in these three studies were 46% ($n = 25$), 52% ($n = 30$) and 49% ($n = 49$); all higher than the expected value of 20–30%.

In the small randomised trial (based on giving thalidomide to patients who had already responded to standard chemotherapy), the median survival was 11.7 ($n = 49$) and 8.7 ($n = 43$) months in the thalidomide and placebo arms respectively; a substantial difference for this disorder.

However, a large double-blind placebo-controlled phase III trial (724 patients) of thalidomide vs placebo was conducted. The results showed no evidence of an effect. The median survival was 10.1 and 10.5 months in the thalidomide and placebo arms respectively. The one-year survival rates were 37% and 41% respectively.

Some treatments that appear effective in phase II studies are shown to be ineffective when tested in a phase III trial. An example is shown in Box 4.3. Conversely, there are likely to be some effective treatments that are not investigated further because phase II data were not supportive of an effect.

Phase II studies provide valuable initial information about a new treatment. 'Positive' results are used to underpin the justification for a larger trial, thereby making such a trial more likely to be funded, and for it to obtain approval from a regulatory authority and ethics committee. Even if the data were negative, indicating that there is unlikely to be a beneficial effect, it is useful to have this information because it means valuable subjects and resources have not been wasted by having a larger study.

4.8 Summary points

• Phase II studies are a useful way of obtaining preliminary information about a new intervention in a relatively small number of subjects.
• There are several different designs, including those that have a comparison arm. The design should be specified before the trial commences.
• Subjects should be monitored closely, especially for side-effects.
• The results of phase II studies are generally descriptive, focusing on the size of the effect of the new intervention and the 95% confidence interval.

- The characteristics of patients entered into the trial should be described in sufficient detail.
- Careful consideration should be given to interpreting the data from randomised phase II studies that contain a control arm, particularly if they produce positive results.
- The decision to conduct a larger, confirmatory trial should depend on several factors: efficacy, safety and feasibility.

References

1. Simon R, Wittes RE, Ellenberg SS. Randomized phase II clinical trials. *Cancer Treat Rep* 1985; **69**:1375–1381.
2. Scher HI, Heller G. Picking the winners in a sea of plenty. *Clinical Cancer Research* 2002; **8**:400–404.
3. Steinberg SM, Venzon DJ. Early selection in a randomised phase II clinical trial. *Statist Med* 2002; **21**:1711–1726.
4. Lee JJ, Feng L. Randomized phase II designs in cancer clinical trials: current status and future directions. *J Clin Oncol* 2005; **23**:4450–4457.
5. Rubinstein LV, Korn EL, Friedlin B *et al.* Design issues of randomised phase II trials and a proposal for phase II screening trials. *J Clin Oncol* 2005; **23**:7199–7206.
6. Wieand HS. Randomized phase II trials: what does randomisation gain? *J Clin Oncol* 2005; **23**:1794–1795.
7. Machin D, Campbell M, Fayers P, Pinol A. Sample size tables for clinical studies. 2nd edn. Blackwell Science, 1997.
8. Tan, SB & Machin, D. Bayesian two-stage designs for phase II clinical trials. *Stat Med* 2002; **21**:1991–2012.
9. A'Hern R. Sample size tables for exact single-stage phase II designs. *Stat Med* 2001; **20**:859–866.
10. Fleming TR. One-sample multiple testing procedure for phase II clinical trials. *Biometrics* 1982; **38**(1): 143–151.
11. Simon R. Optimal two-stage designs for phase II clinical trials. *Controlled Clinical Trials* 1989; **10**:1–10.
12. PASS (Power Analysis and Sample Size software): http://www.ncss.com/pass.html
13. nQuery: http://www.statsol.ie/html/nquery/nquery_home.html
14. Lee S-M, Buchler T, James L *et al.* Phase II trial of carboplatin and etoposide with thalidomide in patients with poor prognosis small-cell lung cancer. *Lung Cancer* 2008; **59**(3):364-8.
15. Lee SM, Rudd RM, Woll PJ *et al.* Two randomised phase III, double blind, placebo controlled trials of thalidomide in patients with advanced non-small cell lung cancer (NSCLC) and small cell lung cancer (SCLC). *J Clin Oncol* 2008; **26** suppl; abstr 8045.

CHAPTER 5

Design of phase III trials

A randomised controlled trial (phase III trial) should provide enough evidence to warrant a change in practice. There are various types of randomised trials, and the design depends on the objectives. The principles of minimising bias and confounding, and the advantages of blinding are presented in Chapter 1.

5.1 Objectives of phase III trials

The main objective of a phase III study is usually based on **efficacy** or **safety**, or both. Box 5.1 summarises common trial objectives in relation to two interventions. The method of sample size estimation depends on the appropriate objective. Defining what is 'better' or 'worse' depends on the outcome measure used. Common efficacy endpoints are mortality, occurrence of the disease of interest, further advancement (progression) of a disease being treated, cure or relief of chronic symptoms, or change in lifestyle or behaviour. In conducting equivalence or non-inferiority trials, the aim is usually to show that two interventions have a similar efficacy, but one is safer, more cost-effective or easier to administer.

There are also **bioequivalence drug trials**, in which two forms of the same drug, for example, produced using a new method or a different formulation, are compared, rather than two different drugs. All that is required is to determine that a similar amount of drug is taken into the body (i.e. similar bioavailability), and this can be done using a biochemical marker or other surrogate. A completely new trial with one of the common true efficacy endpoints such as mortality or disease cure is unnecessary. If bioequivalence is demonstrated, it is assumed that there would be the same effect on a true endpoint.

5.2 Types of phase III trials

Common trial designs are illustrated in Figure 5.1. There are several key considerations:
- What are the interventions?
- What is the main objective and corresponding outcome measure?
- Do the researchers or subjects know which intervention has been allocated (**single** or **double blinding**)?

A concise guide to clinical trials, First edition. By A. Hackshaw. Published 2009 by Blackwell Publishing, ISBN: 978-1-4051-6774-1.

***

Box 5.1 Trial objectives

Comparing two interventions, A and B

(B could be the standard treatment, placebo or no intervention)

Superiority	A is more effective than B
Equivalence	A has a similar effect to B
Non-inferiority	A is not less effective than B (i.e. it could have a similar effect or be better)

'Effect' is associated with any primary trial endpoint, such as death, or occurrence or recurrence of a disorder

Equivalence and non-inferiority trials are usually conducted when the new intervention is expected to have fewer side-effects, be more cost-effective or be more convenient to administer.

***

- Are there independent groups of subjects, where each subject receives only one treatment (**parallel groups** or unpaired data), or does each subject receive all the trial treatments (**crossover trial** or paired data)?

Most trials have **parallel groups**: each group of subjects receives only one intervention. They are used when treatments have long-lasting effects, such as life-threatening disorders, or for disease prevention or cure. For chronic disorders, where the desired outcome is relief of symptoms rather than disease cure, it is possible to allocate both the new and standard treatment to the same subject in sequence in a **crossover trial**. This design is also used for bioequivalence trials (page 57). Instead of randomly allocating subjects to treatment arms, the ordering of treatments is random, so that a similar number of people given treatment A first are given treatment B first. If at least three treatments are evaluated, a latin square design could be used. The strength of a crossover study is that there are essentially identical treatment groups: each subject is his/her own comparison.

Occasionally, it is possible to administer the two interventions at the same time (**split-person design**). For example, in dentistry, in comparing the effect of two types of fissure sealants on future caries risk, one sealant method could be applied to the left side of the mouth and the other sealant to the right side (called a **split-mouth design**). In medicine, a new topical cream for psoriasis could be evaluated by being applied to one arm and a standard cream applied to the other arm.

Crossover designs have limitations. There should be no **residual (carryover) effect** from the first treatment that influences the response to the second treatment, because this could make it difficult to compare them and distinguish their effects reliably. To minimise this problem, a sufficiently long **washout period** is required – a length of time between the two trial treatments when neither are given. Deciding how long the washout period needs to be depends

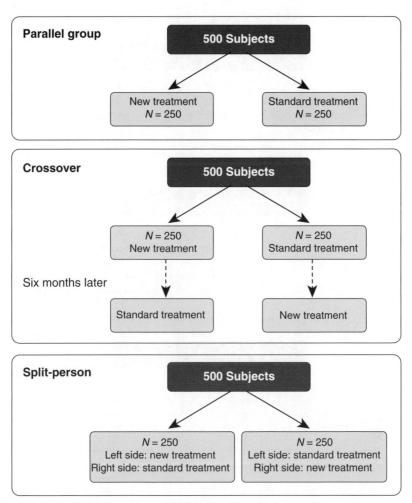

Figure 5.1 Illustration of phase III trial designs using unpaired (parallel) or paired data (crossover or split-person). The solid arrows indicate where the randomisation process takes place.

on the aetiology of the disorder of interest and the pharmacological prop-erties of the trial treatments. Also, the extent of the disorder should reverse back to what it was at baseline after the washout period, i.e. the subject is not cured after the first treatment. In crossover studies, there may also be a **period effect**, in that the ordering of the treatments matters: people who have A then B respond differently to those who have B then A. This can be allowed for in the statistical analysis. If there is uncertainty over the strength of the carry-over effect, or period effect, it may be preferable to use a standard two-arm trial.

Several different treatment combinations or several doses of the same drug can be evaluated in three or more arms (Figure 5.2). A special case of a

Comparing different interventions

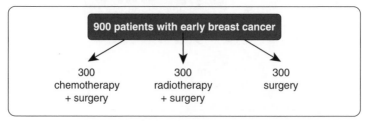

Comparing different doses

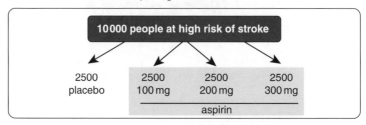

Comparing two new interventions with a control (Factorial)

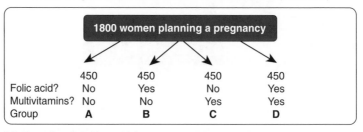

Figure 5.2 Examples of multi-arm trials.

multi-arm study is a **factorial trial**. There are two new interventions, and each is to be compared with a control arm. This is an efficient design because it avoids having two separate two-arm trials, which would mean many more trial subjects in total. There are two distinct contexts; one in which the treatments should not interact with each other, and the other in which an interaction is expected. An interaction occurs if the combined effect of A and B differs from what would be expected by combining the effects seen when A and B are given separately (see page 107). To examine an interaction effect the trial would have to be larger than if no interaction were assumed. Figure 5.2 shows an example of a trial that evaluated folic acid and a multi-vitamin combination for preventing neural tube defects among pregnant women. The following comparisons could be made:

- B + D vs A + C (is folic acid effective?)
- C + D vs A + B (are multivitamins effective?)

- D vs B (is folic acid plus multivitamins better than folic acid alone?)
- D vs C (is folic acid plus multivitamins better than multivitamins alone?).

A factorial trial can only be conducted if both interventions can be given to a subject, and safety should be monitored closely, especially in the combined arm.

Allocating individuals or groups of individuals to the trial groups

Most trials involve randomising individual subjects to different arms, and this is the preferable approach. However, there are occasions when this is not practical, and groups of subjects are randomised instead. An example would be a trial to determine whether a new educational programme aimed at teenagers could reduce their prevalence of smoking and alcohol drinking. The trial could compare the programme with no intervention (control). If children were randomised within the same school to either the programme or control, the effect of the programme could be diluted because children will mix with each other and share their experiences of the programme. Also, the children would have to be separated out to deliver the programme to some and not others, and this may have practical difficulties. An alternative is to randomise schools. All children in one school receive the new programme and all those in another school become the control group. Several schools would be randomised in this way, and it is often a more practical way of delivering both interventions. This is called **cluster randomisation** or a **cluster randomised trial**. Both the sample-size calculation and statistical analysis at the end of the trial should allow for this type of design (see page 109). Data is still obtained from each trial subject.

5.3 Choosing outcome measures

There is some flexibility in the choice of outcome measures in phase II studies, including surrogate endpoints (see page 17). This is done on the understanding that a subsequent, larger trial will use a true endpoint. In phase III trials the main outcome measure needs to be chosen carefully and well defined so that the trial objectives are met, and the results persuade health professionals to change practice. For many trials, the choice of endpoint will be easy, for example death, the occurrence or recurrence of a specific disease, or a change in habits. The main endpoint should be clinically relevant to both the trial subject and the researcher.

When a trial is not blind, the endpoint should be chosen such that the lack of blinding has a minimal effect, because knowing which treatment is received could affect the value of the outcome measures (page 13). The main endpoint should therefore ideally be an **objective**, rather than a **subjective**, measure. Possible examples of objective measures are some blood values, radiological measurements (such as from an X-ray or CT scan) and physiological measurements (such as motor function). If a trial is double-blind, neither objective nor subjective measures should be affected, so either could be used. Many subjective measures are those reported by the subject, such as pain level or health-related quality of life.

Below are possible endpoints in a randomised trial of a flu vaccine in the elderly to prevent flu, presented on page 92:[1]

- Self-reported flu-like symptoms, using a questionnaire completed by patients
- Serological evidence of the flu virus, i.e. an increase in antibodies against influenza detected in a blood sample
- Diagnosis by a clinician after the patient presented with flu-like symptoms
- Hospital admission for respiratory disease (not used in the trial[1]).

All are valid outcome measures, though they have their strengths and limitations.

'Self-reported' flu is easy to measure because there is no need for a clinical assessment by a clinician or a blood test. Patients complete a questionnaire at home and send it to the co-ordinating centre where the responses are examined and subjects are classified as having flu or not according to a set of criteria. However, it is a **subjective measure** that may have wide variability, which could mask a moderate treatment effect. If patients are not blind to treatment they could easily affect this type of outcome measure. Those given the vaccine may be less likely to report fever and headaches, because they think that these symptoms are unrelated to flu. While, those given placebo may be more likely to report these symptoms, which may be unrelated to flu. This bias would make the vaccine seem effective when it is not, or to over-estimate the effect.

'Serological evidence' is an **objective measure**, which should be unaffected by a lack of blinding. However, there will be some individuals who have evidence of the flu virus in their blood but may not feel unwell enough to go to their doctor, or are unaffected, so the clinical importance of this endpoint is uncertain. This measure also involves taking a blood sample, which needs to be stored appropriately and analysed in a laboratory, both of which have a cost implication.

'Diagnosis by clinician' is perhaps in between the previously mentioned subjective and objective measures. It might be considered clinically important because these are the people who have felt so unwell that they decided to go to their doctor. They are more likely to seek medication to relieve their symptoms, go to hospital for respiratory problems, or die from flu. The clinician uses standardised criteria to help classify patients as having flu or not, but this still requires some judgement. Again, knowing whether the patient had the vaccine or placebo could affect the clinical diagnosis of flu, in a similar way to the self-reported outcome.

'Hospital admission for respiratory disease' would be associated with the more severely affected patients. It might be less affected by a lack of blinding. However, it relies on the trial researchers being notified of all admissions of the trial participants. This endpoint can also be used to evaluate the financial costs to the health service provider.

Determining which is the best outcome measure needs careful thought. One of the reasons for having a public health vaccination programme in the elderly is to reduce the morbidity and mortality caused by acquiring the flu virus, and examining hospital admission would address this directly. However, because the proportion of elderly people who are admitted to hospital for flu-related respiratory disorders is low, a large trial is needed in order to see a sufficient number of admissions to be able to conclude reliably that the vaccine had an effect. Serology and diagnosis by clinician are perhaps the most appropriate and complementary endpoints. One is objective, while the other indicates the impact on part of the health service. There are situations when no single end-point is ideal. The choice of outcome measure will also depend on the aim of the trial, the disorder of interest, the interventions being tested, and whether it would change practice.

5.4 Composite outcome measures

While some trial endpoints are associated with the occurrence of a single event, others consist of several events combined into one; called a **composite endpoint**. An example comes from trials of primary or secondary prevention of cardiovascular disease that have evaluated statin therapy using an end-point with four components: fatal or non-fatal coronary heart disease, or fatal or non-fatal stroke. Composite endpoints avoid having to deal with several separate outcome measures at the same time, and it increases the number of events, making it easier to detect a treatment effect, if it exists, and to achieve statistical significance.[#] Figure 5.3 is a hypothetical example, in which it is assumed that Treatment A has a similar effect for each of the events (the point estimates for the relative risk are similar), but on their own the events are not statistically significant (the 95% confidence interval line includes the no effect value of 1.0). The composite endpoint is statistically significant, because it is based on more events. The events have equal 'weight', for example it is assumed that subjects consider a non-fatal myocardial infarction as important as non-fatal stroke. Where this is unlikely to be true, it is possible to give different numerical weights to each constituent event.

A limitation of composite endpoints is that a new intervention could work for some but not all of the constituent events. Figure 5.4 shows the results from a randomised trial in patients with angina, comparing invasive with medical therapy.[2] The composite endpoint result is clearly driven by hospital admission for acute coronary syndrome. There is no clear evidence of a benefit associated with death or non-fatal myocardial infarction: the 95% confidence intervals contain 1.0, i.e. there is a possibility of no real difference between the

---

[#]Statistical significance and confidence intervals are presented in Chapter 7.

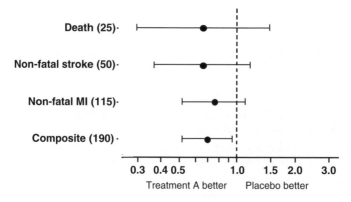

Relative risk (95% confidence interval)

Figure 5.3 Hypothetical results of a trial of treatment A versus placebo. The number of events is shown in brackets for each endpoint. The relative risk is the proportion of patients who had an event with Treatment A divided by the proportion on placebo. A relative risk of 1.0 (the no-effect value) means that Treatment A and placebo had the same effect. MI: myocardial infarction.

interventions. It may then be difficult to make claims of effectiveness. A solution is to present analyses in the final report based on the composite and each of the constituent events, and discuss the implications of the results.

When using composite endpoints the first occurrence of any of the events is used. This is because the clinical management of the patient may affect the risk of any subsequent event that occurred after the first event, making it difficult to distinguish the effects of the interventions.

Defining a composite endpoint should be done at the start of the trial, i.e. in the protocol, with clear justification for the constituent events. If the trial

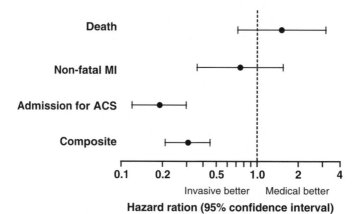

Hazard ration (95% confidence interval)

Figure 5.4 Randomised trial comparing invasive with medical therapy for patients with angina. The hazard ratio is the risk of having an event in 'invasive therapy' divided by the risk in 'medical therapy', at any time point (discussed in reference 2). MI: myocardial infarction; ACS: acute coronary syndrome.

results are to be used for licensing, the validity of the composite endpoint should be first verified with the regulatory body (e.g. the US Food and Drug Administration) to ensure it will provide the necessary evidence needed for a successful application. However, difficulties may still arise if differences in the composite endpoint appear to be the result of differences in only one of the constituent endpoints. See Montori *et al.* for a concise discussion.[2]

5.5 Having several outcome measures (multiple endpoints)

Having one primary endpoint is often easier with trials of life-threatening disorders such as coronary heart disease, stroke or cancer, in which a common endpoint is mortality, or occurrence or recurrence of a disorder. However, for many chronic diseases there could be a range of possible endpoints and the temptation exists to include most or all of them in a trial. A new intervention may appear to work for some endpoints but not others, making it difficult to interpret the results of the trial. It may also be viewed as a 'fishing expedition', i.e. deliberately choosing many endpoints in the hope that at least one will show an effect. Having multiple endpoints increases the chance of finding a spurious effect, unless the sample size is increased. Given these considerations, it is preferable to focus on one or two primary endpoints, and stipulate at the start of the trial that these will be used to determine whether practice should change. The other endpoints should be treated as secondary outcome measures, used to provide further information about the effect of the intervention on the disorder. If there are two or more primary endpoints the sample-size calculation and statistical analysis may need to allow for this (see page 115).

5.6 Fundamental information needed to estimate sample size

The sample size for a phase III trial is based on directly comparing two or more groups of subjects.

Information needed to calculate sample size

- Expected effect in the new intervention group
- Expected effect in the control (comparison) group
- Significance level (usually 5%, at the two-sided level*)
- Power (usually 80% or 90%).

*One-sided if the trial objective is to examine whether the new treatment is not worse than the control (i.e. non-inferiority), or that it can only be better

---

Deciding how many subjects to recruit is an important aspect of design for a phase III trial, because these studies aim to change practice. If there are too

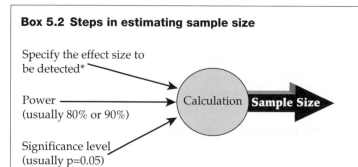

Box 5.2 Steps in estimating sample size

Specify the effect size to be detected*

Power (usually 80% or 90%)

Significance level (usually p=0.05)

Calculation → Sample Size

*The effect size depends on the type of outcome measure used (see Chapter 7):
- 'Counting people' – two proportions (for relative risk or risk difference)
- 'Taking measurements on people' – standardised difference (for the difference between two means)
- 'Time-to-event data' – two survival rates at a specific time point, or two median survival times (for hazard ratio)
- Any other statistic that is associated with making comparisons

few subjects, a clinically important difference may be missed. If there are too many subjects, resources could be wasted and a delay may occur in offering a superior treatment to future patients. There are three elements that determine sample size (Box 5.2):

Expected effect size

The term 'effect size' is used to compare an endpoint between two trial groups. It could be summarised by a relative risk, risk difference, hazard ratio or difference between two means. These are presented in Chapter 7 (Sections 7.1 to 7.4). The magnitude of the effect size could be based on previous knowledge, for example, from a phase II trial, or one that is judged to be associated with a minimum clinically important effect. For equivalence and non-inferiority trials a range is specified within which it is possible to say that a new intervention has a similar effect (**maximum allowable difference**, see page 69).

Level of statistical significance

Statistical significance is often set at 5% (0.05): the results will be determined to be statistically significant at this level.[#] This is the chance of finding an effect when in reality one does not exist, so the conclusion of the trial would be wrong. If there are multiple primary endpoints (e.g. three) a lower level can be specified (e.g. 0.017, calculated as 0.05/3). In conducting superiority trials a two-sided level is typically used, usually at the 5% level, to allow the new intervention to be better or worse than the control group. Sometimes, a more

---

[#]Some textbooks refer to statistical significance as α, or Type I error.

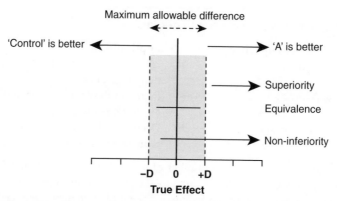

Figure 5.5 Illustration of three possible comparisons between Treatment A and a control group. The effect could be the difference between two percentages, for example, the percentage of patients who recover from the disorder. 'D' is the maximum allowable difference. The true difference could be any point on the horizontal bars.

stringent 1% level is specified. One-sided tests should only be used when the new intervention can only be better. For equivalence trials, it is important to exclude a possible difference that is more extreme than the maximum allowable difference in either direction (Figure 5.5). The total significance level can be set at 2.5% or 5%. For non-inferiority studies, the aim is to reliably exclude the possibility that the new treatment is worse than the control group, and therefore a one-sided level of 2.5 or 5% is usually specified.

Power

Power can be interpreted as the chance of finding an effect of the magnitude specified, if it really exists. A high power is required, such as 80 or 90%, used by most trials[#]. However, if the trial will be unique or expected to have a significant impact on health practice, researchers may choose 95% power, though this greatly increases sample size and the feasibility of this needs to be considered.

Power

At the end of the trial the following statement needs to be true:
'The observed difference of 50% vs 65% is statistically significant at the 5% level'

↓

There needs to be an 80% chance of being able to make this statement (80% power), if there really is a difference of at least 15 percentage points.

Changing any of these three elements affects sample size (Box 5.3).

[#]Some textbooks refer to 100 minus power as β, or Type II error.

Box 5.3 Why sample size would get larger

Sample size goes up when:		Implications:
Effect size gets smaller	$\longrightarrow$	Harder to detect small differences than large ones
Power goes up	$\longrightarrow$	Increases the chance of picking up the effect if it really exists
Significance level goes down	$\longrightarrow$	Decreases the chance of saying there is an effect when there is no true effect

What is also important is the number of events when the endpoint is 'taking measurements on people' or 'time-to-event' data. While it is expected that large studies should have many events, a large study with few events can have low power to detect small or moderate treatment effects.

5.7 Method of sample-size calculation

To determine the method of sample-size calculation, one option from each of the three following features should be chosen:
- The type of outcome measure used:
  - Counting people
  - Taking measurements on people
  - Time-to-event data
- What is being sought when comparing the two interventions:
  - Superiority
  - Equivalence
  - Non-inferiority
  - Factorial (if looking for an interaction)
- Having separate patient groups or one group receives all treatments:
  - Parallel group
  - Crossover (split-person).

There are several methods.[3–6] Free or commercially available software are also available,[3,7–9] and statistical software packages have sample-size facilities.[10–13] It is, however, worth working with a statistician when designing the trial and estimating sample size.

Type of outcome measure

When the outcome measure is based on counting people the two expected percentages (or risks) are specified for each trial arm. The sample size for a difference depends on the actual value of the percentages. For example, the sample size comparing 10 vs 15% is 1372 subjects, but for 50 vs 55% it is 3130, even though the difference is 5 percentage points in both cases.

When taking measurements on people the expected mean value of the outcome measure in each group, and the standard deviation must be specified, and the **standardised difference** calculated. The standard deviation is assumed to be similar between the groups.

$$\text{Standardised difference} = \frac{\text{Mean value in Group 1} - \text{Mean in Group 2}}{\text{Standard deviation of the measurement}}$$

The effect size is therefore defined in terms of the number of standard deviation units. An advantage of working with the standardised difference is that it has no specific unit of measurement, and it does not depend on the actual values of the two individual means (unlike 'counting people' measures). This means that the same standardised difference associated with any comparison yields the same sample size.

For time-to-event data, there are various methods to estimate sample size depending on how the effect size is specified. For example:
• The expected survival rate at a specific time point in each trial arm
• The expected survival rate in the control arm, and the expected hazard ratio
• The expected median survival time in each arm, with additional information on the length of the recruitment and follow-up periods.

What is being sought when comparing the two interventions?

When examining two interventions, it is necessary to determine whether they are likely to have a different or similar effect. To show that one treatment is better than another is relatively easy. Only the two expected percentages in each trial arm, or standardised difference, is required in the sample-size calculation. To show that two interventions have a similar effect, an acceptable degree of difference needs to be specified, i.e. the **maximum allowable difference** (or **equivalence range** or **equivalence limit**). Figure 5.5 illustrates three possible scenarios. There is no rule for determining the maximum allowable difference (D). It could be a third or half of what is considered a clinically important effect. As long as the effect size is within this equivalence range, it can be concluded that the two interventions have a similar effect.

Equivalence studies aim to show that the observed effect size and its confidence interval is within a relatively narrow range around the no-effect value (e.g. page 108), but not more extreme than D at either end. For example, if the trial endpoint is the percentage of patients alive at one year, two treatments could be compared by taking the difference between the two percentages (new treatment minus standard). Specifying a value of $D = 10\%$ means that the corresponding sample size should produce a confidence interval for the difference that is completely within $\pm 10\%$ to conclude equivalence (if they really have a similar effect).

For non-inferiority studies, only one end of the confidence interval for the effect size should not exceed D. It allows for the possibility that one treatment is actually better than the other, or that they are similar. Using the above example, this simply means that the sample size estimated for this study design should not produce a confidence interval that has a lower limit that exceeds −10%.

Specifying a value for D is sometimes difficult. For example, if the main endpoint is the cure rate for a disorder at one year and it is expected that a new intervention has the same rate as standard therapy (say 40%), what maximum allowable difference could be taken to conclude equivalence? If the trial is designed to detect a true cure rate within ±1 percentage points, it is possible to be very confident that the new treatment has an equivalent effect. However, obtaining such a narrow confidence interval requires a very large study (75 000 subjects, 80% power and two-sided level of 5%). Specifying that the cure rate must be within a wide range of ±15 percentage points, requires a much smaller trial (330 subjects). However, with a possible cure rate of 25% (40 minus 15%) it will probably not be considered by many health professionals that the new treatment has a similar effect. The value for D is therefore a balance between something that is not too small and something that would persuade the health community to change practice, but feasible within a trial. In the example, perhaps D between 5 and 10 percentage points would be acceptable. A similar principal applies to non-inferiority trials.

Factorial trials are often used to examine superiority, and the sample size for the comparison of each main effect can be treated as if it were from a two-arm trial. However, if the researcher wishes to have enough statistical power to look at the interaction the sample size needs to be increased.

Having separate subject groups (parallel) or one group receiving all treatments (crossover)

Generally, crossover trials need approximately half the number of subjects required for parallel group trials, because there is not as much natural variation as having two separate groups of people; each subject acts as his/her own control. It becomes easier to detect treatment effects by greatly reducing variability, so a smaller number of subjects is needed.

5.8 Examples of sample-size calculations

Table 5.1 shows sample sizes based on 'counting people' endpoints in a superiority trial. It gives an indication of how large a phase III trial needs to be, and how sample size depends on the effect size and power. A similar observation is seen for 'taking measurements on people', or time-to-event data. Choosing a sample size that seems feasible in a certain timeframe and *then* specifying the effect size is not a good approach, because the effect size is probably quite different from reality. Trials should set out to detect the minimum clinically important difference. The sample-size estimate only reflects the contributing

Table 5.1 Examples of sample sizes when the outcome measure is based on 'counting people'. The table shows the total number of trial subjects required for a two-arm parallel-group study.*

% expected with the outcome in the control arm	% expected with the outcome in the new intervention arm	Effect size % (difference)	Power	
			80%	90%
5	10	5	870	1160
	15	10	280	380
	20	15	150	200
	25	20	100	130
10	15	5	1370	1840
	20	10	400	530
	25	15	200	270
	30	20	120	160
50	55	5	3130	4190
	60	10	780	1040
	65	15	340	450
	70	20	190	250

*rounded to the nearest 10

assumptions. If the assumptions are unrealistic, the size of the trial will be too small or too large.

Sample sizes for non-inferiority and equivalence studies are larger than superiority trials, because the effect size associated with the maximum allowable difference is usually smaller than what is considered to be a clinically important effect, or the significance level is smaller than the 5% level (Box 5.3). Specifying a large maximum allowable difference to minimise the number of trial subjects should be avoided because it could produce results that are too imprecise, making it difficult to draw reliable conclusions.

Table 5.2 provides examples of sample-size descriptions that could be used in a grant application or trial protocol. It is useful to justify the specified effects in each trial arm, or the effect size, using previous studies or unpublished evidence. Box 5.4 shows two quick formulae for estimating sample size for superiority trials.

5.9 The importance of having large enough trials, and specifying realistic effect sizes

There is nothing precise about a sample-size estimate. It provides an *approximate* size of the trial. It does not matter if one set of assumptions yields 500 subjects but another gives 520, because this represents only an extra 10 subjects per trial group. What is more important is whether 500 or 1000 subjects are needed. There is always some guesswork involved in specifying the assumptions for sample size, particularly when determining the effect size, which is often quite different from what is observed at the end of the trial.

Table 5.2 Hypothetical sample size descriptions that could be used in a grant application or protocol.

Type of outcome measure	Trial objective	Description (The numbers in bold are the ones used in the calculation to produce the sample size.)
Counting people	Superiority	The proportion who develop flu by 5 months is **10%**. It is expected that the flu vaccine would decrease the incidence to **5%**. To detect a difference of 10 vs 5% requires a trial of 580 subjects in each arm (vaccine and placebo), with **90%** power and **two-sided test** of statistical significance at the **5%** level. Total trial size is 1160 subjects.
Counting people	Equivalence	The proportion of patients who normally respond to standard treatment is **55%**. Drug A is expected to have an equivalent effect. A maximum allowable difference of **±10** percentage points will be used to conclude Drug A and standard treatment are equivalent. To show this requires a trial of 520 subjects per arm, with **80%** power and **2.5%** level of statistical significance, **two-sided test**. Total trial size is 1040 patients.
Counting people	Noninferiority	The proportion of patients who usually respond to treatment is **50%**. Therapy B should not have a response rate that is much worse than this. A maximum allowable difference of up to **–5** percentage points (i.e. a response rate not below 45%) would indicate that Therapy B is not inferior. To show this requires a trial with 1570 patients in each arm, with **80%** power and **one-sided test** of statistical significance at the **2.5%** level. Total trial size is 3140 patients.
Taking measurements on people	Superiority	The mean loss in body weight using conventional diets is 5 kg. It is expected that Diet K would be associated with a mean weight loss of 8 kg. The standard deviation of weight change is 4 kg. To detect a standardised difference of **0.75** [(8–5)/4] requires a trial of 40 patients in each arm with **90%** power and **two-sided test** of statistical significance at the **5%** level. Total trial size is 80 subjects.
Taking measurements on people	Noninferiority	A pain killer, with fewer side-effects, is expected to not be worse than standard treatments. The usual mean pain score on a visual analogue scale (VAS) is 75 mm, with a standard deviation of **40 mm**. The new drug should not be worse than 85 mm (i.e. the mean VAS needs to be lower than this), corresponding to a maximum allowable difference of **10 mm**). To show this requires a trial of 340 patients in each arm, with **90%** power and **one-sided test** of statistical significance at the **2.5%** level. Total trial size is 680 patients.
Time-to-event data	Superiority	The median survival associated with the standard treatment is **18** months. Therapy A is expected to have a median survival of **24** months. It is expected that the recruitment of patients would take **36** months, after which there will be **12** months of follow up (i.e. the total length of the trial is 4 years). To detect a difference of 18 vs 24 months requires 315 patients in each treatment arm, with **80%** power and **two-sided test** of statistical significance at the **5%** level. Total trial size is 630 patients.

Box 5.4 Quick formulae for estimating sample size for superiority trials (two-sided 5% level of statistical significance)

	Example
'Counting people':	
Expected percentage on new treatment $= P2$	0.20 (20%)
Expected percentage on standard treatment $= P1$	0.30 (30%)
Number of subjects in each arm $=$	80% power, $N = 296$

$$\frac{[P1 \times (1 - P1) + P2 \times (1 - P2)]}{(P2 - P1)^2} \times F$$

90% power, $N = 390$

'Taking measurements on people':

Expected mean value on new treatment $= M2$	7.0
Expected mean value on standard treatment $= M1$	5.0
Standard deviation $= SD$	3.5
Standardised difference $= \Delta = (M2 - M1)/SD$	0.57
Number of subjects in each arm $= F \times 2/\Delta^2$	80% power, $N = 50$
	90% power, $N = 65$

$F = 8$ for 80% power
$F = 10.5$ for 90% power

The smaller the true effect size, the larger the study needs to be, because it is more difficult to distinguish between a real difference and random variation. Consider mortality as the main endpoint in a trial comparing Drug A and placebo, with 100 subjects per group. If the one-year death rate is 15% for Drug A and 20% for placebo, the effect size, expressed as a risk difference, is five percentage points[#] – this represents only five fewer deaths among 100 subjects given Drug A. It is not easy to tell whether this difference is real, i.e. a true treatment effect, or simply due to chance. There could just happen to be five fewer deaths in this trial arm. However, if the death rates were 5% versus 40%, this would be a difference of 35 percentage points, or 35 fewer deaths among 100 subjects on Drug A, and this is unlikely to be due to chance.

In a trial 10 times as big as the one above (i.e. 1000 subjects per arm), a comparison of one-year death rates of 15% and 20% is still five percentage points, but it is based on 150 versus 200 deaths; a difference of 50 deaths.

[#]'five percentage points' is a better way of describing the effect than '5%' when comparing two percentages. It avoids the possible confusion over whether the death rate for Drug A is $5\% + 15\% = 20\%$ rather than 5% greater than 15%, which would be $1.05 \times 15\% = 16\%$.

Again a difference as large as this is unlikely to be due to chance, and likely to be due to a real treatment effect of Drug A.

In the past, large treatment effects were often sought for many disorders including cardiovascular disease and cancer, because new treatments at the time were being compared with placebo or minimal treatment. Significant improvements in treatments and prevention have since occurred, and these are the current standard of care against which new treatments now need to be compared. This means that moderate or even small effects are often now expected, requiring larger study sizes.

A very large study should give a clear answer to the research question. Resources may be saved by conducting a small trial, but a clinically important difference between two treatments may be missed because the result is not statistically significant (see page 113), when in fact there is a real effect, but the study is too small to detect it. This can occur when the true effect is smaller than that specified in the sample size calculation. When this happens, it is difficult to make reliable conclusions. This is why it is important to try to detect the smallest clinically worthwhile effect, with 80 or 90% power, in order to have an appropriately sized study. For example, if the aim is to only recruit about 130 subjects, an effect size (standardised difference) of 0.5 could be specified (Box 5.4). But if the real effect size were 0.2, 790 subjects are needed; a smaller trial is likely to miss this.

When the trial objective is to examine equivalence or non-inferiority, the new treatment is sometimes expected to be associated with fewer side-effects. It is sometimes useful to ensure that the target sample size is also large enough to reliably detect a difference in adverse events.

5.10 Reasons for increasing the sample size

The sample-size estimate assumes that there will be a measure of the trial endpoint on every subject at the end of the trial. This is not possible in many trials because some subjects will withdraw from the trial (**patient drop-outs** or **patient withdrawal**, see page 118). However, a certain proportion of drop-outs can be allowed for. If the estimated sample size were 500 subjects and 10% were expected to withdraw, the trial would aim to recruit about 556 patients, because 556 less 10% is $500[500/(1 - 0.10)]$.

Some trials have one or more **interim analyses**, i.e. early looks at the data, with the aim of possibly stopping the trial early if a large treatment effect is found, or the effect observed is so small that there is unlikely to be a clinically important effect if the trial continued (see page 122). When this is planned, the sample size can be increased to allow for having several analyses.

Other reasons for increasing sample size could be to allow for having two or more primary endpoints (page 115), unequal randomisation (page 83), subgroup analysis (page 119), or to examine an interaction between two new treatments in a factorial trial (page 107).

5.11 Other considerations in designing phase III trials

Once the main trial endpoints and estimated sample size are determined it is useful to assess the feasibility of recruitment, the number of recruiting centres that might be needed and the duration of the trial. This will provide an idea of the financial costs and how the study could be conducted.

An issue that may arise is whether subjects could simultaneously enter more than one clinical trial. Alternatively, subjects finishing one trial may be asked to enter a subsequent trial soon after. Neither is encouraged because it might be difficult to separate out the different treatment effects. If there are situations when this might occur it is necessary to ensure that it will still be possible to address the research question of each trial, and that no bias or confounding has been introduced. Researchers of both studies should be aware of this. The worst scenario is where there is a serious imbalance in the arms of the second trial (Figure 5.6). This can be avoided by ensuring that subjects who enter Trial 2 are **stratified** at the time of randomisation (see Chapter 6) for the allocated treatment arm from Trial 1.

In some disease areas, usually uncommon disorders, it is possible to conduct a **phase II/III** trial. Here, a phase III randomised trial is designed and conducted, but an assessment of efficacy is made early on (e.g. after a quarter of subjects have been recruited), similar to an analysis in a phase II trial. Sometimes, the study is temporarily halted so that further patients are not recruited and treated until the phase II assessment is complete. The purpose is to judge whether the new treatment is unlikely to be effective, so the trial could stop early. It could also be used to investigate several new treatments

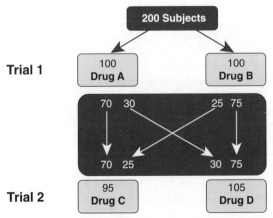

Figure 5.6 Hypothetical situation where subjects can enter one trial after another and confounding of treatments has occurred. The Drug C group is dominated by patients who previously had Drug A, and the Drug D group is dominated by patients who previously had Drug B.

simultaneously to decide which merited continued investigation. The results based on the interim data are not published, and should only be seen by the trial statistician and an independent **Data Monitoring Committee** (see page 179). As well as being an efficient use of subjects (those in the phase II part can be included in the full phase III trial), a practical advantage of not having completely separate phase II and III trials is that the 'seamless' approach does not need two separate clinical trial applications, approval from two ethics committees and two set-up procedures at centres. This reduces the time taken to evaluate a new intervention.

5.12 Summary

• Phase III trials are considered the 'gold standard' for evaluating a new intervention

• They should be designed to be sufficiently large to provide reliable evidence

• There are several types of objectives: superiority, equivalence and non-inferiority

• The main outcome measure should be relevant to the trial subjects, researchers and those who may benefit in the future

• The methods for estimating sample size depend on the type of outcome measure, the trial objective and whether there are separate groups of subjects, or subjects get all treatments.

References

1. Govaert TME, Thijs CTMCN, Masurel N *et al.* The efficacy of influenza vaccination in elderly individuals. *JAMA* 1994; **272**(21):1661–1665.
2. Montori VM, Permanyer-Miralda G, Ferreira-Goonzales I *et al.* Validity of composite end points in clinical trials. *BMJ* 2005; **330**:594–596.
3. Machin D, Campbell M, Fayers P, Pinol A. *Sample Size Tables for Clinical Studies*, 2nd Edn. Blackwell Science, 1997.
4. Pocock S. *Clinical Trials: A Practical Approach.* John Wiley & Sons, Ltd, 1983.
5. Julious SA. Tutorial in biostatistics. Sample sizes for clinical trials with Normal data. *Stat Med* 2004; **23**:1921–1986.
6. Jones B, Jarvis P, Lewis JA, Ebbutt AF. Trials to assess equivalence: the importance of rigorous methods. *BMJ* 1996; **13**:36–39.
7. Power and Sample Size calculation. DuPont WD, Plummer WD. http://medipe. psu.ac.th/episoft/pssamplesize/
8. PASS (Power Analysis and Sample Size software): http://www.ncss.com/pass. html
9. nQuery: http://www.statsol.ie/html/nquery/nquery_home.html
10. STATA: http://www.stata.com
11. MINITAB: http://www.minitab.com/
12. SAS (Statistical Analysis Software): http://www.sas.com/
13. SPSS (Statistical Package for the Social Sciences): http://www.spss.com

CHAPTER 6

Randomisation

Randomly allocating individuals, or groups of individuals, to two or more interventions is the key design feature of all phase III clinical trials. It should ensure that the characteristics of individuals are similar between the trial groups (i.e. **minimises confounding**), and **minimises bias** (Chapter 1, page 12). This is achieved by ensuring that trial staff entering each subject, or the subjects themselves, cannot predict the treatment allocation (Box 6.1). It is also expected that the intervention arms have similar numbers of subjects, unless otherwise specified.

For relatively small trials, say less than 100 subjects, there are simple randomisation methods that can be carried out by hand, but for large multi-centre trials it is preferable to use a computer. By removing all human influence from the random allocation process, possible biases are minimised. There are different methods of randomisation, and their strengths and limitations should be considered.

6.1 Simple randomisation

In its most basic form, randomisation can be done by simply throwing a coin: if Heads, give Treatment A; if Tails, give Treatment B. However, the coin could be thrown until a preferred treatment allocation is obtained for a particular subject. Using a **random number list** is better (the numbers 0 to 9 in a random order). This can be obtained from statistical tables or random number generator functions within software such as Microsoft Excel.

Table 6.1 provides an example of a random list of 12 numbers for allocating subjects to two interventions. The first and second subjects recruited receive A, the third receives B, and so on. In the table, the number of subjects in each arm is identical (six in each). With large trials (several hundred or several thousand subjects) simple randomisation should produce similarly sized groups. However, it is possible to get a noticeable imbalance when the trial size is small (say <30 subjects), just by chance. Among the first six subjects in Table 6.1, two received Treatment A and four received Treatment B. Extending this to a trial of 20 subjects, there could be 13 on one arm and 7 on the other, simply because of the ordering of the random numbers. Although the allocation process has been truly random, having unequal treatment groups could affect the

A concise guide to clinical trials, First edition. By A. Hackshaw. Published 2009 by Blackwell Publishing, ISBN: 978-1-4051-6774-1.

Box 6.1 Randomisation

- Randomisation produces treatment groups that have similar characteristics other than the trial intervention
- The only systematic difference between the trial arms is the treatments given
- Any observed difference in the trial endpoints should be due to the effect of the treatment and not to any other factors.

Randomness = unpredictability

What is important is that the next treatment allocation cannot be predicted by the person entering the subject.

---

statistical analysis when making comparisons between groups – it can reduce statistical power. Furthermore, it would be unfortunate if there were fewer subjects on the new intervention arm, the arm of most interest.

To ensure that treatment groups have a similar size, **random permuted blocks** can be used. A block size, which must be divisible by the number of interventions is specified. For two treatments the block size is often four or six, sometimes eight or greater. In every consecutive group of four subjects there are equal numbers in the trial arms. Each treatment should appear at least twice in each block. Table 6.2 illustrates one way of using random permuted blocks. Each random number determines the allocation for the next four subjects, not one subject as before.

For three treatments, the block size needs to be divisible by three, such as six or nine. With a block size of nine, the numbers 1 to 9 could be randomly ordered:

- 1–3 give Treatment A
- 4–6 give Treatment B
- 7–9 give Treatment C.

For four treatments, as in 2×2 factorial trials, the block size could be 8 or 12. Using a block size of 12, and a random ordering of the numbers 1 to 12:

- 1–3 give Treatment A
- 4–6 give Treatment B
- 7–9 give Treatment C
- 10–12 give Treatment D.

A limitation of random permuted blocks is that the allocation for the last subject in the block can be predicted if the previous allocations are known. This

Table 6.1 Random number list used to allocate 12 subjects to Treatment A or B.

Random number list	4	1	6	5	8	5	2	3	0	7	9	2
Subject identifier*	1	2	3	4	5	6	7	8	9	10	11	12
Treatment allocation	A	A	B	B	B	B	A	A	A	B	B	A

If random number is: 0–4: give Treatment A; 5–9: give Treatment B
*This is also the ordering in which subjects are recruited

Table 6.2 Random number list used to allocate 12 subjects to Treatment A or B using a block size of four. The first three random numbers are 4, 1 and 6 (from Table 6.1).

Random number list		4				1				6		
Subject identifier*	1	2	3	4	5	6	7	8	9	10	11	12
Treatment allocation	B	A	B	A	A	A	B	B	A	B	B	A

If random number is: 1 – AABB; 2 – BBAA; 3 – ABAB; 4 – BABA; 5 – BAAB; 6 – ABBA (ignore random numbers 0, 7, 8 and 9)
*This is also the ordering in which subjects are recruited

can be avoided by having a mixture of block sizes, so that the person randomising the subjects is unaware of whether the next subject is in a block size of, say, four or six. For double-blind trials, knowing the block size should not matter.

For crossover or split-person trials, where each subject receives all interventions in sequence or at the same time, the ordering of the treatments needs to be randomised, so that a similar proportion of subjects receive 'A' or 'B' first. This is achieved by randomly allocating subjects to receive either 'A followed by B' or 'B followed by A' (Table 6.3). In a split-person design, patients are randomised to receive 'A to the left side and B to the right side' or 'B to the left side and A to the right side'.

Simple randomisation is easy to implement by hand or by computer, but it ignores important prognostic baseline factors that can affect the value of the trial endpoint. This should not matter for large trials, because getting large chance imbalances in these factors will be rare. However, for small or moderately sized trials, these differences could affect the trial results. If, for example, the percentage of patients with severe disease happened to be 20% on Treatment A and 35% on Treatment B, this difference may partly explain a difference in the trial endpoints, by making B appear worse. Although imbalances can be allowed for in the statistical analysis, the adjusted results could still be viewed with caution. It is better to avoid large imbalances during recruitment. The two following methods of randomisation achieve this (**stratified randomisation** and **minimisation**).

Table 6.3 Random number list used to allocate 10 subjects to Treatment A and B in sequence in a crossover trial.

Random number list	4	1	6	5	8	5	2	3	0	7
Subject identifier*	1	2	3	4	5	6	7	8	9	10
Treatment allocation	AB	AB	BA	BA	BA	BA	AB	AB	AB	BA

If random number is: 0–4: give Treatment A then B; 5–9: give Treatment B then A
*This is also the ordering in which subjects are recruited

6.2 Stratified randomisation

Stratified randomisation attempts to guarantee balance for some important **stratification factors**. These could include age, gender and severity of disease, but the number and type of factors will vary between trials, and should be selected carefully. Recruiting centre may also be included if subjects are spread over a wide geographical region, and there are clear differences in local practice. In surgical trials, a stratification factor could be surgeon, in which case it may not necessary to also include centre. A stratification factor should not have levels with few expected subjects. For example, if disease severity (moderate and severe) were included, but <1% of patients are expected to fall in the 'severe' category, it would not be worth including this factor in the randomisation process.

Stratification involves using simple randomisation *within each level of the factor*. For categorical variables, such as gender, centre or disease severity (mild, moderate, severe), the factor levels are already defined. For continuous measurements, such as age, weight and many blood values, the range must be converted into categories.

Table 6.4 illustrates stratified randomisation using age alone. A random number list is generated for each age group. For example, the first subject, who is aged 52 years, is randomised using the random number list under '50–59' years, and the fourth patient, aged 68 years, is randomised under the '60–69 years' list. Block sizes of four or more can be used to ensure that the number of subjects is similar between the treatment arms. With two stratification

Table 6.4 Illustration of stratified randomisation using one factor (age). Twelve patients have been randomised using the appropriate strata for their age.

Age group				
40–49 years				
Random number list*	4	1	6	5
Treatment allocated	A	A	B	B
Subject identifier*	3	8	9	11
Age (years)	48	40	43	41
50–59 years				
Random number list	0	7	4	1
Treatment allocated	A	B	A	A
Subject identifier*	1	2	6	12
Age (years)	52	55	53	58
60-69 years				
Random number list	9	6	3	1
Treatment allocated	B	B	A	A
Subject identifier*	4	5	7	10
Age (years)	68	65	65	61

If random number is: 0–4: give Treatment A;
5–9: give Treatment B
*This is also the ordering by which subjects are recruited

Table 6.5 Illustration of stratified randomisation using two factors, age and gender.

Gender	Age group (years)											
	40–49				50–59				60–69			
Male												
Random number list	4	6	2	5	7	5	3	1	4	1	5	9
Treatment allocated	A	B	A	B	B	B	A	A	A	A	B	B
Female												
Random number list	0	7	4	1	8	3	7	4	4	8	9	1
Treatment allocated	B	A	A	B	B	A	B	A	A	B	B	A

If random number is: 0–4: give Treatment A; 5–9: give Treatment B

factors, for example age and gender, simple randomisation is performed within each combination of the factor levels (Table 6.5). There is a random number list in each cell of the table.

Stratified randomisation is generally a good way of balancing important prognostic factors, and can be relatively easy to do by hand. Problems arise when one or more stratification factors have many levels, or several factors are specified. While two to four factors may be necessary, sometimes far too many are used.

In a real example of a double-blind treatment trial of lung cancer, comparing placebo with a drug called Tarceva, the following stratification factors were included:

- Quality of life performance status (three groups)
- Smoking status (two groups)
- Tumour stage (two groups)
- Recruiting centre (50 centres).

A randomisation list is needed for *every* combination of these four factors, i.e. $3 \times 2 \times 2 \times 50 = 600$ lists. Randomising patients would be cumbersome to do by hand, and there are likely to be many cells with only one or two patients, particularly if the trial size is not large. There could be more cells than patients, leading to a chance imbalance in the number of patients in the trial arms, or in one or more of the stratification factors.

After the first 301 patients were recruited out of a target sample size of 664, by chance alone the first patient randomised in each of several centres was allocated to Tarceva, and many centres had only recruited one patient. There were 168 patients in the Tarceva arm, 26% greater than that in the placebo arm ($n = 133$). Although a difference of this magnitude would have a minimal effect on the statistical analysis, it can give the false impression that the randomisation process did not work properly. As expected, the size of the difference diminished as more patients were randomised within each of the stratification factors. The limitations of stratified randomisation can be largely overcome by careful selection and justification of the stratification factors, or by using a method called minimisation.

6.3 Minimisation

Minimisation also aims to ensure balance between the treatment groups for pre-specified prognostic factors. The treatment allocation for the first few subjects (e.g. 20) can be made using a single random number list (as in simple randomisation). However, the allocation for each subsequent subject depends on the distribution of the stratification factors among those who have already been randomised, and not using random numbers. Minimisation is also referred to as **dynamic allocation**.

Table 6.6 illustrates one method of minimisation. It is based on a hypothetical trial in which 20 patients have already been recruited, and a random number list used. The distribution of each factor is obtained. The next (21st) subject, who is 45 years old, female and with moderate disease, needs to be randomised. The total for Arm A is less than for Arm B so the 21st patient is allocated to Arm A. If the total for B was lower, the subject is allocated to Arm B. If the totals are identical, allocation can be made using a random number list. This method of minimisation only considers the balance in the categories which apply to the patient being randomised, but there are more sophisticated methods that consider the overall balance across all categories.

An advantage of minimisation is that it can cope easily with any number of stratification factors, including those with many levels, but it is best implemented using a computer program. Though this should not encourage researchers to use as many as they can.

It is sometimes argued that minimisation is not truly random because the next allocation is predictable and could be susceptible to bias. This can be partly overcome by using a high probability of allocating to the next treatment. In the example, this would mean that the 21st patient has an 80 or 90% chance of being allocated Arm A, rather than a 100% chance; allocation to Arm A is not completely certain.

Table 6.6 Illustration of a simple method of minimisation using three stratification factors.

| Factor | Level | Number of subjects | | 21st subject |
		Arm A	Arm B	
Age	40–49 years	4	3	Age 45
	50–59	4	2	
	60–69	2	5	
Gender	Male	5	5	
	Female	4	6	Female
Disease status	Mild	3	3	
	Moderate	2	4	Moderate
	Severe	4	4	
Sum		10	13	

Sum for A is less than sum for B, so 21st subject receives Treatment A

For single centre studies, minimisation should not be used in case the person allocating the treatments is aware of the allocations. However, for multi-centre trials it is difficult for trial staff in one centre to know of the treatment allocations from all centres and all stratification factors, and therefore correctly guess the next allocation. Given that the randomisation process means unpredictability (Box 6.1), minimisation is an acceptable method for trials with at least two centres.

Methods of randomisation

- Simple randomisation (with or without a specified block size)
- Stratified randomisation (with or without a specified block size)
- Minimisation

– A block size of k means that after every k subjects have been recruited, the number of subjects in each treatment arm is the same
– Stratified randomisation and minimisation ensures the trial arms are well balanced for specified important prognostic factors
– In simple and stratified randomisation, the allocation of one subject to the trial groups is independent of the allocation of all other subjects
– In minimisation, the allocation of a subject depends on the previous allocations.

6.4 Unequal randomisation

Most trials aim to have a similar number of subjects in each treatment arm (**equal** or **1:1 randomisation**). Sometimes, more subjects are required in one arm (**unequal randomisation**), usually the new intervention, such as in the ratio 2:1. This may be because more reliable data is needed on the effects of the new treatment (e.g. side-effects). Also, subjects may be more likely to participate in a trial if they have a 2 in 3 chance of getting a potentially more effective treatment, rather than a 50% chance.

For the same sample size, the statistical power associated with comparing the results of two trial arms decreases as the number of subjects in each arm becomes more unequal. However, the loss in power is only considered unacceptable if the ratio exceeds 3:1. In the example of the lung cancer trial on page 81, the imbalance is noticeable to the eye (168:133), but the ratio (1.3:1) would not mean a great loss of power in the statistical analysis. To avoid loss of power, unequal randomisation can be allowed for in the sample size calculation by having a larger study size.

6.5 Which method of randomisation to use?

The choice of randomisation method depends on the size of the trial, the number of stratification factors, and availability of a computerised randomisation

Table 6.7 Crude guide to choosing the randomisation method in a two-arm trial.

Size of trial (total number of subjects)	Number of stratification factors		
	None	Few (all with a few levels)	Many (some with many levels)*
Small (<50)	Simple	- Stratified - Minimisation	Minimisation
Moderate (50–199)	Simple	- Stratified - Minimisation	Minimisation
Medium (200–999)	Simple	- Stratified - Minimisation	Minimisation
Large (>1000)	Simple	- Simple - Stratified - Minimisation	- Stratified - Minimisation
Very large (>10 000)	Simple	- Simple - Stratified - Minimisation	- Simple - Stratified - Minimisation

*or a few factors, of which some have many levels

program. The randomisation process is often performed by hand in small trials, because the development and maintenance costs associated with a computer program are not worthwhile. Table 6.7 is a crude guide to how trial size and number of stratification factors might influence the randomisation method used.

The aim of achieving balance in important prognostic factors justifies using methods such as stratified randomisation or minimisation. However, having trial arms with equal numbers is not a necessary outcome of randomisation, chance variation should produce arms with slightly different sizes.

For crossover or split-person studies, subject characteristics and prognostic factors are, by design, identical between treatment arms because each subject acts as his/her own control. Simple randomisation should therefore be acceptable. Stratified randomisation might be considered to ensure that, for example, a similar proportion of males and females have Treatment A followed B, and vice versa.

When stratification factors are used, it is recommended that adjustment is made for the factors in the statistical analysis (using the multi-variate methods in Box 7.11, page 114). This might seem counter-intuitive because these factors were used specifically to ensure balance. The reason is that the randomisation process has been 'restricted' by incorporating these stratification factors, compared with simple randomisation. Adjusting for them in the analysis can increase the precision of the results (narrower confidence interval), though the effect size does not usually change much. Both the unadjusted and adjusted effect sizes (and 95% confidence intervals) could be presented for the main endpoint.

6.6 Eligibility

Inclusion and exclusion criteria (**eligibility list**) are always defined (see page 11). When potential subjects are identified, this list is examined to ensure that the subject is suitable for the trial. The subject can then be randomised after giving consent. The trial interventions should be administered soon after the allocation has been made. The eligibility list for each subject can be filed in the recruiting centre so that it can be examined during a monitoring visit (see page 179).

Some trials have a long eligibility list, which may make it difficult to recruit the target sample size in a timely fashion. A cut-off for each criterion must be specified, but there should be some degree of flexibility. When a subject's value is just outside of the range, a judgement could be made whether to randomise or not. For example, if the required age range is 50 to 80 years, but a potential subject is aged 49 years and was eligible in relation to all other factors, it would be reasonable to randomise them; the age is very close to the cut-off. A subject aged 35 years should probably not be randomised. The decision to randomise will depend on the importance of the criteria used, and how close to the limit for inclusion the subject falls.

It is useful to have a **screening log** in each participating centre, which records each eligible subject approached, and whether they declined to participate in the trial and why. This could be used to identify problems with recruitment.

6.7 Randomising in practice

The logistical aspects of randomly allocating subjects varies according to the size of the trial and the resources available. Trials co-ordinating within dedicated clinical trials units or established research departments should already have the computing expertise to implement any type of randomisation method requested. Outside such settings, methods such as simple or stratified randomisation (with one or two stratification factors) can be done by hand. A statistician or computer programmer sometimes produces the randomisation list, which can be created using a random number generator available in many software packages. When allocating subjects, it is often best for a computer program to read off the list rather than a person (e.g. trial co-ordinator), because it avoids human error, which could occur when using stratified randomisation or minimisation. This is especially so for large trials.

Tossing a coin for all trial subjects should be avoided because bias cannot be detected, and there is no formal record of a randomisation list until after the subject has been randomised. A randomisation list or minimisation process can show the regulatory authorities, or the sponsor's auditor, that treatment allocation has been properly conducted. However, if a computer randomisation program is used and there is a rare occasion when the system is not functioning, tossing a coin is a simple solution at the time. Other methods of

Table 6.8 Randomisation lists using simple randomisation in two trials; an unblinded trial (surgery vs chemotherapy) and a blinded trial (aspirin vs placebo).

	Unblinded trial			Blinded trial		
Random number	*Treatment allocation*	*Patient number*	*Treatment allocation*	*Pack code*	*Subject number*
3	Surgery	1	Aspirin	M1001	1
7	Chemotherapy	2	Placebo	M1002	2
8	Chemotherapy	3	Placebo	M1003	3
0	Surgery	4	Aspirin	M1004	4
1	Surgery	5	Aspirin	M1005	5
3	Surgery	6	Aspirin	M1006	6
8	Chemotherapy	7	Placebo	M1007	7
2	Surgery	8	Aspirin	M1008	8
4	Surgery	9	Aspirin	M1009	9
5	Chemotherapy	10	Placebo	M1010	10

Allocation: Treatment A if random number is 0–4 and Treatment B if 5–9

randomising subjects include sealed envelopes, each one containing the next allocation, based on a random number list (e.g. surgical trials).

For blind trials, the randomisation list will not show the interventions. The list of subjects and their actual treatment is not revealed until the end of the trial. Only the randomisation programmer and trial statistician should have access to this list during the trial because neither have direct contact with subjects or staff who recruit and manage subjects. The programmer and statistician cannot, therefore, influence the treatment allocation, or the trial outcome measures. The randomisation list visible to other trial staff only contains a treatment code, sometimes called medication or 'med' number, or 'pack code'. This code could be created by the trial co-ordinating centre, or the drug supplier, but it is essential that the supplier labels the drugs correctly. Named trial staff can obtain the actual allocation for a particular subject when, for example, there is a serious adverse event, and knowing what trial treatment was given will help (see page 182).

Table 6.8 is an example of a randomisation list using simple randomisation. Working down the list, the first patient (ID code 1) is allocated to surgery, the second patient receives chemotherapy and so on. In the blinded study, trial staff or anyone else involved in randomisation would only see the pack code and patient identifier. The first patient randomised would be sent drugs labelled M1001 by the supplier. The supplier would need to ensure that the aspirin packets are labelled M1001, M1004, M1005 etc., and the placebo packets are labelled M1002, M1003, M1007.

Multi-centre trials usually have a trial co-ordination centre with dedicated staff. Subjects are randomised after recruiting centres contact the trial centre (usually by telephone or fax) who, after checking eligibility, uses a computer randomisation program to inform the centre of the treatment allocation. For international trials, where subjects could be recruited at any time of the day in relation to the co-ordinating centre, it is often impractical to have 24-hour trial staff. Instead, an internet randomisation system, or automated telephone service with voice recognition, can be used, neither of which require direct contact with trial staff. These systems can be expensive to set up and require expert IT staff to develop and maintain. Central randomisation has the advantage that the treatment allocation is performed by someone who has no direct contact with the subject, thus minimising the potential for bias.

6.8 Checking that the randomisation process worked: examining baseline characteristics

All trial reports should have a table comparing the baseline characteristics between the interventions. The aim is to show that randomisation produced similar arms, indicating that the results are valid and unlikely to be explained by any factor other than the treatments being tested. If the characteristic is based on 'taking measurements on people', the mean (or median) values should be similar between the groups. If based on 'counting people', the proportions should be similar.

P-values (discussed in Chapter 7) are sometimes provided for the baseline comparisons. They indicate whether an observed difference could have arisen by chance, assuming that the distribution of the factor in one group is identical to the distribution in another group. However, it is inappropriate to examine baseline differences in this way.[1] P-values test whether a baseline factor for ≥ 2 groups came from the same distribution, but this is known to be true because the randomisation was made from the same group of subjects in the first place. Reporting and interpreting p-values for baseline characteristics should therefore be avoided. Randomisation should produce small imbalances. What matters is whether the size of the difference is likely to distort the comparison of the treatments.

Table 6.9 shows the baseline characteristics in a trial comparing different methods of inhaled sedation during oral surgery among anxious children, in

Table 6.9 Baseline characteristics and main outcome measure of a trial comparing methods of inhaled sedation during oral surgery among anxious children.[2]

	Air N = 174	Nitrous oxide N = 256	Nitrous oxide + sevoflurane N = 267	P-value for the difference between the three groups
Baseline characteristic				
Males (%)	47%	50%	39%	0.03
Mean age (years)	9.1	9.5	9.6	0.11
Mean body weight (kg)	36.3	37.8	37.7	0.50
Level of anxiety (mean score)	5.6	6.1	6.0	0.01
Main trial endpoint				
Percentage of children who completed surgery	54%	80%	93%	<0.001

All children received intravenous midazolam

which p-values for baseline factors were reported.[2] The main endpoint was whether the dentist was able to complete the surgery. While most factors were similar between the groups, there appeared to be a difference in gender and anxiety level, indicated by a p-value <0.05. There was a lower percentage of males in the 'nitrous oxide plus sevoflurane' group, and children who received air tended to have lower anxiety levels. Instead of focusing on the p-value, the extent to which the outcome measure of the trial could be affected by these imbalances needs to be considered, as well as plausibility.

The trial results could be affected if gender or anxiety levels were associated with the chance of completing treatment. For example, the percentage of males in the 'nitrous oxide plus sevoflurane' group was eight percentage points lower than in the group who received air (39 vs 47%). Gender could have an effect if males are less likely than females to complete surgery, because the lower completion rate in the 'air' group (54%) could be due to the higher proportion of males. This might not be plausible. Furthermore, it is unlikely that such a large treatment effect (93 vs 54%, a difference of 39 percentage points) could be explained by a difference of only eight percentage points. Similarly, the average anxiety level in the 'nitrous oxide plus sevoflurane' group was 0.4 units higher than that in the 'air' group. This could affect the endpoint if children with higher anxiety levels are more likely to complete surgery, but this again is questionable, and a difference of 39 percentage points is unlikely to be due to a difference of only 0.4 units. Despite an apparent statistically significant difference in these two factors, the treatment effect is unlikely to be materially affected. The trial results are valid.

When the number of subjects in a trial is very large, even small and unimportant baseline differences could be highly statistically significant. It would be incorrect to conclude that the randomisation process failed. When observed differences appear large enough to matter, checks can be done. First, it must be established that subjects were correctly allocated from the randomisation list, by looking for human error or error in the programming code. Second, selection or allocation bias needs to be eliminated as a possible cause (probably not as necessary for double-blind trials). For example, screening logs within centres could be examined to determine whether certain eligible subjects were not randomised to one of the trial arms, or were withdrawn soon after randomisation, but not included in the trial. Whatever these checks show, there are statistical methods that can allow for differences in baseline characteristics when analysing the main trial endpoints, (the multi-variate methods on page 114). However, it is best to ensure similarity during recruitment.

6.9 Summary

- The three commonly used methods of randomisation are: simple and stratified randomisation, and minimisation.
- There is no perfect method of randomisation; one may be more appropriate than another for a particular trial.

- The choice of method can depend on the trial size, the number of important prognostic factors that need to be allowed for, and logistical and resource issues.
- Randomisation does not need to produce trial arms with equal numbers, and the distribution of baseline characteristics needs to be only similar, not identical, between the groups.

References

1. Senn SJ. Testing for baseline balance in clinical trials. *Stat Med* 1994; **13**:1715–1726.
2. Averley PA, Girdler NM, Bond S, Steen N, Steele J. A randomised controlled trial of paediatric conscious sedation for dental treatment using intravenous midazolam combined with inhaled nitrous oxide or nitrous oxide/sevoflurane. *Anaesthesia*, 2004; **59**:844–852.

CHAPTER 7

Analysis and interpretation of phase III trials

Randomised controlled trials aim to change practice so their data needs careful analysis and interpretation. Phase III trials always compare at least two intervention groups. The data can be interpreted using the following fundamental questions:

- Is there a difference? Examine the **effect size**.
- How big is it?
  - What are the implications of conducting a trial on a **sample** of people (**confidence interval**)?
- Is the effect real?
  - Could the observed effect size be a **chance finding** in this particular trial (**p-value** or **statistical significance**)?
- How good is the evidence?
  - Are the results **clinically important**?

An **effect size** is a single quantitative summary measure used to interpret clinical trial data, and to communicate the results. It is obtained by comparing a trial endpoint between two intervention arms. Types of effect sizes depend on the outcome measure used: 'counting people', 'taking measurements on people' or 'time-to-event' data (see Chapter 2), which also determines the method of statistical analysis. This chapter presents the commonly used analyses, but there are more complex ones that are appropriate when necessary.

7.1 Outcome measures based on counting people

Consider a trial that evaluated the effect of an influenza vaccine in the elderly (Box 7.1).[1]

What are the main results?
Each percentage (or proportion) indicates the **risk** of developing flu. For example, the risk of being diagnosed with flu by the family doctor after five months in the placebo arm is 3.4%. The **effect size** is either the ratio (**relative risk** or **risk ratio**), or the difference (**absolute risk difference**) between the two risks. Using the results in Box 7.1, these are interpreted as follows:

A concise guide to clinical trials, First edition. By A. Hackshaw. Published 2009 by Blackwell Publishing, ISBN: 978-1-4051-6774-1.

Box 7.1 Example: Phase III trial of the flu vaccine in the elderly[1]

Location: 15 family health practices in the Netherlands

Subjects: 1838 men and women aged $\geq$60 years

Design: Double-blind placebo-controlled randomised trial

Interventions: A single flu vaccine or placebo (saline) injection

Main outcome measures: The proportion who developed flu up to 5 months after the injection; diagnosed by (i) serology or (ii) family doctor

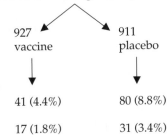

1838 individuals aged $\geq$60 years

927 vaccine   911 placebo

Flu diagnosis five months later By serology	41 (4.4%)	80 (8.8%)
By family doctor	17 (1.8%)	31 (3.4%)

- Relative risk = 4.4% ÷ 8.8% = 0.50: Vaccinated people are half as likely to develop serological flu than those given placebo, after five months
- Risk difference = 4.4% − 8.8% = −4.4%: Among vaccinated people, 4.4% fewer cases of serological flu are expected compared to those given placebo. Alternatively, in 100 vaccinated subjects there could be 4.4 fewer cases than in a group of 100 given placebo. (The minus sign indicates fewer cases.)

The **comparison**, or **reference group** must always be made clear.[#] They usually receive standard treatment, placebo or no intervention. It is insufficient to say 'Vaccinated subjects are half as likely to develop serological flu'. What is correct is: 'Vaccinated subjects are half as likely to develop serological flu *compared with placebo subjects*'. If the reference group were vaccinated subjects, the relative risk would be 2.0 (8.8% ÷ 4.4%): placebo subjects are twice as likely to develop serological flu as vaccinated subjects. The risk difference would be +4.4% (8.8% − 4.4%): in 100 subjects given placebo there could be 4.4 more cases of serological flu than in a group of 100 vaccinated subjects.

The 'no-effect' value
If the vaccine had no effect, both groups would have the same risk of developing flu. The relative risk (the ratio of the two risks) is one, and the risk

---

[#] It might also be useful to know the actual risk in this group.

difference is zero. These are called the no-effect value. They help interpret confidence intervals and p-values.

Is the new intervention better or worse?
The relative risk or risk difference indicates the magnitude of the effect. Determining whether the intervention is more beneficial or harmful depends on what is measured. 'Risk' implies something bad, but in research it can be used for any endpoint. If the outcome measure is 'positive', for example, the percentage of people who are alive, an increased relative risk (i.e. >1), or positive risk difference (i.e. >0), indicates that the new intervention is more beneficial. However, if the outcome measure is 'negative', such as the percentage of people who have died, an increased relative risk or positive risk difference indicates that the intervention is more harmful.

Further interpretations of risk difference and relative risk
There are other ways to help explain the treatment effect. A risk difference can be converted to **Number Needed to Treat (NNT)**. The risk difference for serological flu is −4.4%, meaning that in 100 vaccinated subjects there were 4.4 fewer flu cases. To avoid one case of serological flu, 23 people need to be vaccinated (100 ÷ 4.4). The NNT is 23 (Box 7.2).

Relative risks of 0.5 or 2.0 are easy to interpret: the risk is half or twice as large as in the reference group. However, values of 0.85 or 1.30 are less intuitive: the risks are 0.85 or 1.30 times as large as that in the reference group. Converting relative risk to a **percentage change in risk** can be useful (Box 7.3): called either a **risk reduction**, or an **excess risk**. From Box 7.1, the relative risk of 0.53 (1.8% ÷ 3.4%) means that the risk of developing clinician-diagnosed flu is reduced by 47% in those who were vaccinated, compared with the placebo group. The no-effect value for a percentage change in risk is zero.

Generally, a relative risk below 2.0 is changed to a risk reduction or excess risk. If above 2.0 it is better left alone, to avoid looking cumbersome. A relative risk of 12 is an excess risk of 1100% ([12 − 1] × 100). It is acceptable to say the risk is 12 times greater, or increased 12-fold.

Box 7.2 Calculating the number needed to treat (NNT) to avoid one affected individual

Risk of developing serological flu*

Vaccine	Placebo	Risk difference	NNT
4.4%	8.8%	−4.4%	23 (100 ÷ 4.4)
0.044	0.088	−0.044	23 (1 ÷ 0.044)

*expressed as a percentage or proportion

Box 7.3 Converting a relative risk to percentage change in risk

Relative risk (RR)	Subtract the no-effect value of 1 (RR − 1)	Multiply by 100 (RR − 1) × 100	
0.85	−0.15	−15%	relative risk reduction (or risk reduction)
1.30	+0.30	+30%	excess relative risk (or excess risk)

A positive sign indicates the risk is increased, compared to the reference group

A negative sign indicates the risk is decreased

Relative risk or risk difference?

Relative risks tend to be similar across different populations, indicating the effect of a new intervention *generally*. They do not usually depend on the underlying rate of disease. A relative risk of 0.5 associated with a flu vaccine means that the risk is halved from whatever it is in a particular population, whether the flu incidence is 1 per 1000, or 20 per 1000. However, risk difference always reflects the underlying rate, and so will vary between populations. It indicates the treatment effect *in a particular population*. As the disease becomes more common, the relative risk is not expected to change much, but the risk difference will increase and the NNT decreases (Table 7.1). An intervention has a greater effect in a population when the disease is common. Because risk difference can vary, relative risk is the most commonly reported effect size. Risk difference could be given in addition.

What are the implications of conducting a trial on a sample of people?

When using a sample of people in a trial to estimate the true effect size among all subjects who could benefit from the intervention, there is uncertainty over

Table 7.1 Relative risk and risk difference according to different underlying disease rates (i.e. in the placebo group).

Risk of flu				
Placebo (per 100)	Vaccine (per 100)	Relative risk	Risk difference (per 1,000)	Number needed to treat
1	0.5	0.50	5	200
2	1.0	0.50	10	100
5	2.5	0.50	25	40
10	5.0	0.50	50	20
20	10.0	0.50	100	10

Table 7.2 Effect size and 95% confidence intervals (CI) associated with comparing two proportions (or percentages).

Outcome measure	Risk of flu		Effect size	
	Vaccine N = 927	Placebo N = 911	Relative risk 95% CI	Risk difference 95% CI
Flu diagnosis by:				
Serology	4.4%	8.8%	0.50 0.35 to 0.72	−4.4% −6.6 to −2.1%
Family doctor	1.8%	3.4%	0.53 0.30 to 0.97	−1.6% −3.0 to −0.1%

how close the observed effect size will be to the true value. This is quantified by a **standard error**, used to calculate a **95% confidence interval** (CI) for a relative risk or risk difference. The basic principle is the same as that for a single proportion or mean (Chapter 4 and Figure 4.1).

95% Confidence interval for a relative risk or risk difference

A range within which the **true** relative risk, or **true** risk difference, is expected to lie with a high degree of certainty. If confidence intervals were calculated from many different studies of the same size, 95% of them would contain the true value, and 5% would not.

Table 7.2 shows the 95% CIs from the flu vaccine trial. The relative risk for serological flu is 0.50 with 95% CI 0.35 to 0.72. The *true* relative risk is thought to be 0.50, but there is 95% certainty, given the results of this trial, that the true value lies somewhere between 0.35 and 0.72. The interval excludes the no-effect value (relative risk of one), so there is likely to be a real effect of the vaccine. The corresponding percentage risk reduction is 50%, and the true value is likely to lie between 28 and 65% (calculation in Box 7.3). The ends of the CI provide a conservative and optimistic estimate of the effect size, and in this example, even a 28% risk reduction may be considered worthwhile. The CI for the risk difference indicates that the true effect could be anywhere between 2.1 and 6.6 fewer cases of flu in every 100 vaccinated people.

There is likely to be a real treatment effect if:

The 95% CI for the relative risk excludes the no-effect value of 1

The 95% CI for the excess risk or risk reduction excludes the no-effect value of 0

The 95% CI for the risk difference excludes the no-effect value of 0

Describing a CI sometimes implies that the true effect lies anywhere within the range with the same likelihood. However, it is more likely to be close to the point estimate used to derive the interval (i.e. the middle) than at the extreme ends. This is an important consideration when the interval just overlaps the no-effect value. With a relative risk of 0.75, and 95% CI 0.55 to 1.03, most of the range is below the no-effect value. The possibility of 'no effect' cannot be reliably excluded because the interval just includes 1.0, but the true relative risk is more likely to lie around 0.75 than 1.0. A treatment effect should not be dismissed completely with this kind of result, because there is a suggestion of an effect.

Could the observed effect size be a chance finding in this particular study?

The observed risk difference associated with serological flu, in the 1838 trial subjects, was −4.4%. But what is of interest is the effect in all subjects that could benefit from the vaccine. If the trial included *every* elderly person ever, might the difference be as large as −4.4%, or even greater, or could there in fact be no difference at all?[#] Could the observed difference of −4.4% be a chance finding in this particular trial, due to natural variation? To help determine this, a **p-value** is calculated. The size of the p-value depends on the difference between the two risks (effect size), the sample size on which each risk is based, and the number of events (i.e. cases of flu).

The p-value for a risk difference of −4.4%, with each risk based on 41/927 and 80/911, is <0.001. Even if there were really no effect (i.e. the true difference were zero), a value of −4.4% could be seen in some studies, just by chance. But how often? The p-value of <0.001 indicates that a difference as large as 4.4% or greater, in favour of either the vaccine or placebo, would occur in less than 1 in 1,000 studies of the same size by chance alone, *assuming* that there really were no effect. The observed effect size (4.4% risk difference) is therefore unlikely to have arisen by chance, and so reflects a real effect. The p-value for clinician-diagnosed flu is 0.035: a risk difference of 1.6% or greater, in either direction, could be seen in 35 in 1,000 studies of the same size, if the true risk difference were zero. The Appendix provides more details.

These are **two-tailed** p-values. Effect sizes of −4.4% or lower (vaccine better than placebo), or +4.4% or greater (placebo better than vaccine), are both assumed to be plausible. Any departure from the no-effect value is allowed for. The p-value is twice as large as a **one-tailed** p-value, which is based on looking only in a single direction. The more conservative two-tailed p-value is reported for most trials, unless there is a clear justification for having a one-tailed value (i.e. the new treatment can only be better).

[#] Or if many other trials were conducted, each with 1838 subjects, would a difference as large as −4.4%, or greater, be observed in many of them, if the vaccine really had no effect?

A new intervention is considered to have a real effect if the p-value is <0.05; a cut-off judged to be sufficient low (see page 112). The result is said to be **statistically significant** (Section 7.6).

How good is the evidence?
The flu vaccine trial was double blind, so the clinician giving the vaccine or placebo injection could not have influenced the allocation. Subjects were also unaware of what they received, so neither group should be no more or less likely to report flu-like symptoms (see page 62). It is possible, therefore, to be confident about the relative risk of 0.50; a large and clinically important effect, which was similar whether flu was determined by serology or clinician diagnosis. In fact, it is close to the effect seen in observational studies. Treatment compliance was not an issue, because the interventions involved a single injection; no subject refused the injection after being randomised.

Relative risk or odds ratio?
A relative risk is easy to calculate. Sometimes, the **odds ratio** is reported. It has some useful mathematical properties used by many statistical methods. 'Risk' and 'odds' are different ways of presenting the chance of having a disorder. Risk is the number with disease out of all subjects, while an odds expresses the number with disease to the number without. If there is one affected subject among n people, there must be $n - 1$ unaffected subjects. So a risk of $1/n$ is the same as an odds of $1/(n - 1)$, or $1 : n - 1$.

When the disease is fairly uncommon (say <20%), relative risk and odds ratio are similar, and so interpreted in the same way (Table 7.3A). However, when the disease is common, they will be noticeably different (Table 7.3B). Odds ratios need careful interpretation because a ratio of two odds is not the same as a ratio of two risks. In Table 7.3B it would be incorrect to interpret the odds ratio as a risk reduction of 75%. The risk has been reduced by 51%, indicated by the relative risk, but the odds in the vaccine group is 0.25 times the odds in the placebo group. This is difficult to explain easily. When a disorder is common, describing an odds ratio as if it were a relative risk could greatly over-estimate the treatment effect; relative risk is preferable.

7.2 Outcome measures based on taking measurements on people

Here, the trial endpoint in each arm is summarised by the mean value and the standard deviation (Chapter 2). An appropriate effect size is the **difference between two means** (or **mean difference**). It often has a Normal distribution, so simple statistical analyses can be used. However, this is not usually the case when taking the ratio of two means, so this tends not to be used.

What are the main results?
Box 7.4 shows an example, and the trial endpoint is body weight.[2] The two groups had a similar weight at baseline: the mean values were 99 and 98 kg in

Table 7.3 Calculation of relative risk and odds ratio using the flu vaccine trial (serological diagnosis).

Table A Incidence of flu is uncommon (from the trial in Box 7.1).

	Developed flu	Did not develop flu	Total
Vaccine group	41 (a)	886 (b)	927 (n_1)
Placebo group	80 (c)	831 (d)	911 (n_2)

Relative risk $= a/n_1 \div c/n_2$ (41/927) $\div$ (80/911) $= 0.50$

Odds of developing flu in the vaccine group $= 41/886$ (a/b)
Odds of developing flu in the placebo group $= 80/831$ (c/d)
The ratio of the odds is (41/886) $\div$ (80/831) $= (a \times d) \div (c \times b) = 0.48$

Table B Incidence of flu is common (hypothetical results).

	Developed flu	Did not develop flu	Total
Vaccine group	300	627	927
Placebo group	600	311	911

Relative risk $= (300/927) \div (600/911) = 0.49$
Odds ratio $= (300 \times 311) \div (627 \times 600) = 0.25$

the Atkins and Conventional diet groups respectively. Each subject's weight at a specified time point is compared with that at the start of the trial (**baseline value**). The analysis is based on 'weight at time T minus weight at baseline', i.e. the *change* in weight.[#] The Atkins diet group lost an average of 6.8 kg from baseline to three months, compared with 2.7 kg in the Conventional diet group.

The effect size (mean difference) is $-6.8 - (-2.7) = -4.1$ kg: the Atkins diet group lost an average of 4.1 kg *more* than Conventional diet subjects. The mean differences in weight change at 6 and 12 months were -3.8 and -1.9 kg respectively. The effect of the Atkins diet seemed largest in the first few months.

The effect size is associated with the *average* change in weight. In the Atkins diet group, some individuals lost more than 6.8 kg, some less, and some could have gained weight or had no weight change. However, the aim is to summarise weight change for a group of people, and not to predict weight change for an individual.

Using the change in endpoint is a simple approach. It is acceptable if the baseline values are similar between the trial arms. If they are not, a **multivariate linear regression** (or **analysis of covariance**) is preferable. This statistical method uses weight at time T as the 'outcome variable', and the baseline value and treatment groups are 'covariates'. This analysis also produces the

---

[#] See footnote to Box 7.4. Results presented in this chapter are associated with people who weighed 100 kg at baseline.

Box 7.4 Example: Phase III trial of the Atkins diet[2]

Location: 3 centres in the United States

Subjects: 63 obese men and women

Design: Randomised controlled trial

Interventions: Atkins diet (low-carbohydrate, high-protein, high-fat) or Conventional diet (low-calorie, high-carbohydrate, low-fat) for up to 1 year

Main outcome measures: Change in body weight (from baseline) at 3, 6 and 12 months after starting the diet

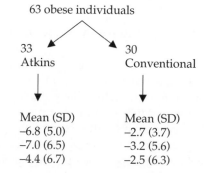

Change in body weight, kg:	Mean (SD)	Mean (SD)
3 months later	−6.8 (5.0)	−2.7 (3.7)
6	−7.0 (6.5)	−3.2 (5.6)
12	−4.4 (6.7)	−2.5 (6.3)

SD: standard deviation; change in body weight = weight at 3, 6 or 12 months minus baseline weight

---

(The published paper was actually based on the *percentage* change in body weight from baseline for each subject. To avoid confusion with percentages used in Section 7.1, the effect of the diets was expressed in kg for the purposes of this chapter, by assuming a baseline weight of 100 kg, close to the mean value in the trial subjects. For example, at three months the reported percentage weight loss in the Atkins group was 6.8%, which is the same as a loss of 6.8 kg in someone who initially weighed 100 kg.)

mean difference in the endpoint at time T between the trial arms, but after allowing for each subject's baseline value.[3]

In judging whether a particular change in weight is clinically worthwhile, a loss of about 7 kg is intuitive, but a weight loss of 1 kg is probably not worthwhile in someone whose initial weight was 100 kg. When trial endpoints are on a restricted scale, the effect size should be interpreted in relation to the scale. For example, pain score is often measured on a visual analogue scale, 0 to 100. A difference in scores of +5 units is a small, perhaps clinically unimportant effect (5/100), but a difference of −30 is not (−30/100).

Table 7.4 Effect sizes, 95% confidence intervals (CI) and p-values from the randomised trial comparing the Atkins and Conventional diets.[2]

Months after baseline	Mean change in weight, kg*		Effect size, kg		
	Atkins N = 33 A	Conventional N = 30 B	Difference in means A − B	95% CI	p-value
3	−6.8	−2.7	−4.1	−6.3 to −1.9	0.001
6	−7.0	−3.2	−3.8	−6.8 to −0.8	0.02
12	−4.4	−2.5	−1.9	−5.1 to +1.3	0.26

*the minus signs simply indicates a reduction in weight compared with baseline (weight at time T minus weight at baseline). [See footnote to Box 7.4]

What are the implications of conducting a trial on a sample of people?

A standard error is estimated using the means and standard deviations (see page 206). It is a measure of uncertainty over how far the observed mean difference is from the true value. The standard error is used to calculate a 95% confidence interval (CI) – a range within which the true mean difference is likely to lie. Three months after starting the diet, the true mean weight loss in the Atkins group is likely to be greater than that in the Conventional diet, by 1.9 to 6.3 kg (Table 7.4). The optimistic estimate of 6.3 kg is a large effect, while the conservative estimate of 1.9 kg may or may not be considered worthwhile. At six months, the effect is less certain because of the wider CI. The lower estimate of 0.8 kg is unlikely to be worthwhile. At 12 months, the 95% CI includes the no-effect value of zero: it is possible that there is no real difference in weight change.

Could the observed effect size be a chance finding in this particular study?

Changes in body weight will vary naturally between people. Some on the Atkins diet will gain weight and some on the Conventional diet will lose weight, and vice versa. A p-value helps determine whether the observed effect size (e.g. −4.1 kg) could be a chance finding that is consistent with this natural variation. At three months the p-value is 0.001 (Table 7.4). An observed effect size as large as −4.1 kg, or greater, could be seen in 1 in 1,000 trials of the same size *if* there were really no difference between the two diets. The effect is therefore unlikely to be due to chance. The benefit of the Atkins diet is likely to be real. However, at 12 months the p-value of 0.26 indicates that a difference of −1.9 kg, or greater, could be seen in 26 in 100 studies of the same size, just due to chance. This is insufficient evidence of a real effect at 12 months.

The p-values in Table 7.4 are **two-tailed**, because the average weight loss could plausibly be greater on either diet. A **one-tailed** p-value should only be used if the Atkins diet can cause weight loss, but not weight gain, which is not true. The p-value of 0.001 at three months is therefore based on a difference in the average weight loss as extreme as 4.1 kg (or greater), in favour of either the Atkins or Conventional diets.

How good is the evidence?

Although an initial weight loss of 4.1 kg might be considered worthwhile, the effect reduced over time probably because more subjects came off the diet (or it took longer for the effect of the conventional diet to be seen). The trial subjects knew which diet they were on, which could affect the results. Atkins diet subjects may have started to exercise more, which led to some of the weight loss. It is difficult to determine what confounders and biases may be present, but a judgement could be made on whether the magnitude of the observed effect could be largely explained by these factors. The mean difference in weight loss at three months was 4.1 kg. Bias or confounding are unlikely to account for all of this. Changes in behaviour, which may influence the trial endpoint, could have been monitored and used to examine whether they could affect the results. Patients could have been asked to record their exercise levels during the trial.

41% of subjects were unavailable for assessment of body weight at the end of the trial (43% Atkins and 39% Conventional). The authors suggest this is largely due to the lack of direct dietary supervision during the trial (subjects were just given written instructions on what to do after an initial meeting with a dietician). This could explain why the effect was greatest in the first few months. The initial large effect might have been maintained if there was more contact with a dietician.

Effect sizes with a skewed distribution

When using the mean difference, calculating CIs and p-values is simple because it is assumed that the difference follows a Normal distribution. If many trials provided a mean difference, the distribution of these differences would appear symmetrical, or bell-shaped (see Figure 2.1, page 20). In practice, the distribution of the endpoint in each trial arm could be examined using a probability plot (Figure 2.3, page 24) to check the Normality assumption.

If the endpoint has a skewed (asymmetric) distribution, applying transformations such as logarithms or square root, may produce a Normal distribution. If the distribution remains very skewed, the difference between two means may not be a good measure of treatment effect. Instead, the **difference between two medians** is better. The calculation of the p-value is based on the ranks of the data, not the actual values, and calculating a 95% confidence interval is more complex.

7.3 Outcome measures based on time-to-event data

In trials with time-to-event data, for example time to death, or time to first stroke, the approach described in Section 7.2 can be used if everyone has had the event of interest. Otherwise, specific methods are available.

Box 7.5 Example: Phase III trial of Herceptin in treating breast cancer[4]

Location: Several centres in the United States

Subjects: 3351 women with early breast cancer and HER2 positive tumours

Design: Randomised controlled trial

Interventions: Standard chemotherapy with or without 1 year of Herceptin

Main events of interest: The number who had a breast cancer recurrence, a new tumour or died.

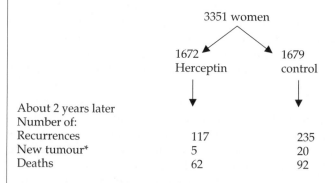

	3351 women	
	1672 Herceptin	1679 control
About 2 years later Number of:		
Recurrences	117	235
New tumour*	5	20
Deaths	62	92

*Not a new breast cancer in the opposite breast

What are the main results?

Box 7.5 is an example of a trial with several time-to-event endpoints.[4] The events of interest were breast cancer recurrence, a new tumour or death. Some women could have more than one of these, for example, a recurrence before dying. The main endpoint is therefore the time to whichever event occurred first, called **disease-free survival** (DFS) in the published paper. Another endpoint was time to death (**overall survival**); see Chapter 2.

Time-to-event data is presented graphically, using a Kaplan–Meier plot (Figure 7.1). DFS rates at specific time points can be read off the graph. For example, at 3 years 87.1% of women in the Herceptin group were alive and free from disease, compared with 75.4% in the control group. Alternatively, 12.9% of women had an event in the Herceptin group compared with 24.6% in the control group; the event rate was approximately halved.

The effect size is the hazard ratio: the risk of an event in one trial arm compared with the risk in the other arm, at the same time point. It can be interpreted in a way similar to relative risk, but is more difficult to calculate by hand because the time to each event needs to be allowed for (statistical software should therefore be used). For a 'negative' event such as death, or disease occurrence, a hazard ratio <1 means that the new intervention is better than the control, because the risk of having an event is lower (i.e. subjects have

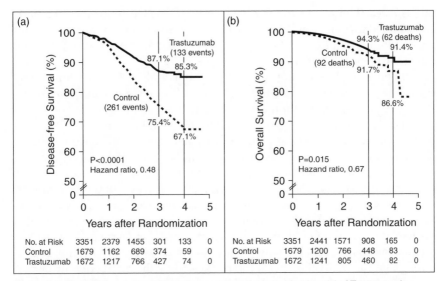

Figure 7.1 Survival curves for disease-free and overall survival for the trial of Trastuzumab (Herceptin) and breast cancer[4] (Note that the vertical axes have been truncated below 50%, so the curves appear more separated than if the full axis had been shown). Reproduced with kind permission from the New England Journal of Medicine.

taken longer to develop the event). For a 'positive' event, such as time until hospital discharge, a hazard ratio >1 indicates benefit, because patients on the new treatment have spent less time in hospital.

In Table 7.5, the DFS hazard ratio is 0.48; the risk of having an event (recurrence, new tumour or dying) in the Herceptin group was about half that in the control group (risk was reduced by 52%). There were also large effects on overall survival (hazard ratio 0.67, or 33% reduction in the risk of dying) and new tumour risk (hazard ratio 0.24, or 76% reduction in risk).

An alternative effect size is the risk difference at a single time point (see also page 105). The absolute risk difference at three years for DFS is 11.7%: 87.1

Table 7.5 Summary results of the trial of Herceptin and breast cancer.[4]

| | Number of events | | Effect size | | |
Endpoint	Herceptin $N = 1672$	Control $N = 1679$	Hazard ratio	95% CI	p-value
Disease-free survival[1]	133	261	0.48	0.39 to 0.59	<0.0001
Overall survival[2]	62	92	0.67	0.48 to 0.93	0.015
New tumour[3]	5	20	0.24	0.09 to 0.64	0.002

1. Time to breast cancer recurrence, new tumour or death, whichever occurred first
2. Time to death from any cause
3. Time to diagnosis of a new cancer, excluding new breast cancers in the opposite breast

If patients did not have an event, they were censored at the date last seen

minus 75.4% (Figure 7.1). Among 100 women given Herceptin, about 12 more are expected to be alive and disease-free three years after randomisation, compared with 100 in the control group. The NNT is eight, i.e. to avoid one patient dying, or having a recurrence or new tumour at three years, eight patients need to be given Herceptin (same calculation as in Box 7.2). The time point should be pre-specified in the protocol to avoid selecting one that appears to show the greatest benefit for the intervention.

A risk difference, while useful to the trial report, has limitations because it is specific to a single time point, and so be affected by chance variation. A hazard ratio is preferable because it compares the whole survival curve between the trial arms. However, it assumes the treatment effect is similar over time: if there is a 25% reduction at three years, there should be a similar reduction at six years.[#] When this is clearly not true, the risk difference at pre-specified time points might be more appropriate. Sometimes, the median survival time (and 95% CI) in each group is reported (if available). Median survival is reliable when many events have occurred continuously throughout the trial, otherwise it can be skewed by the timing of only one or two events. If the distribution of the time-to-event endpoint is 'exponential' (i.e. the event rate is constant over time), the hazard ratio could be estimated by the ratio of the two median survival times. If the median survival times are M1=9 months in the new treatment group and M2=6 months in the control group, the hazard ratio for new vs control is 0.67 (M2/M1).

What are the implications of conducting a trial on a sample of people?

95% confidence interval (CI) for the true hazard ratio (HR) is a range within which the true hazard ratio is likely to lie

95% CI = observed $\log_e$ HR $\pm$ 1.96 $\times$ standard error of the $\log_e$ HR

The results are anti-logged. (The formula for the standard error is not simple, so statistical software should be used to provide the 95% CI; see also page 207.)

The 95% CI for DFS is narrow, so the estimate of treatment effect is precise; i.e. it is likely to lie between 0.39 and 0.59, or a risk reduction between 41 and 61% (Table 7.5). Even the most conservative estimate (41% reduction) is a large effect, so it is possible to be confident that Herceptin is highly beneficial. There were fewer events (i.e. deaths) associated with overall survival, so the

---

[#] Referred to as an assumption of proportional hazards, which appears to hold for most situations.

standard error of the hazard ratio will be larger, contributing to a wider CI: 7 to 52% reduction in risk. The unexpected effect on new tumours seems large (76% reduction in risk), but there is a very wide CI (36 to 91%).

The difference between two survival rates at a pre-specified time point, and 95% CI, can be calculated using the survival rate in the control arm, and the hazard ratio (this is more reliable than using two rates, each of which is affected by chance variability):

Three-year DFS rate in control arm (P) = 75.4% (0.754)

Hazard ratio (HR) = 0.48, 95% CI 0.39 to 0.59

Difference in three-year DFS rate (Herceptin − control) $= e^{HR \times \log_e P} - P$

$= e^{0.48 \times \log_e 0.754} - 0.754 = +0.119$ (11.9%)

95% CI for the difference = 9.2 to 14.2% (by substituting the ends of the CI into the above equation)

Could the observed effect size be a chance finding in this particular study?

The p-values in Table 7.5 are all small: the three effect sizes are unlikely to have arisen by chance, if there really were no effect. The p-value for disease-free survival is particularly small (<0.0001), providing strong evidence that Herceptin is effective.

How good is the evidence?

This large trial has clear results on DFS and overall survival, which are clinically important. Although the trial was not blind it is highly unlikely that these considerable effects could be explained by bias or confounding. The 95% CI for the main endpoint is narrow with a very small p-value. It provides sound evidence that Herceptin is beneficial in women with early breast cancer with HER2 positive tumours. The effect on new tumours is less certain. Although the 95% CI was far from the no-effect value of one, there are only 5 and 20 new tumours in the Herceptin and control arms respectively. Longer follow-up data, or confirmatory results from other trials, are needed before making firm conclusions on this endpoint.

Disease- or Cause-specific survival curves

A new intervention is sometimes expected to only affect the disease of interest. For example, in trials of mammography screening, the aim is to detect breast cancers when they are small, which should only affect breast cancer mortality. Cause-specific survival curves can then be used. An event is 'death from breast cancer', and all other deaths are grouped with people who are still alive or lost to follow up (i.e. censored). Such curves may show a beneficial treatment effect that would otherwise be masked by using all causes of death. In other trials this may not be appropriate. Many oncology trials evaluate toxic anti-cancer drugs, which could cause deaths other than from the cancer of interest. Curves based on overall survival can provide a clearer picture of the treatment effect (see page 28). If cause-specific curves are presented,

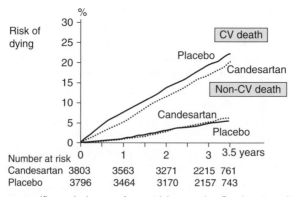

Figure 7.2 Cause-specific survival curves from a trial comparing Candesartan with placebo, and the effect on cardiovascular (CV) death, and other causes of death.[5] The data indicates that Candesartan had a beneficial effect on CV death, but no effect on other causes. Reproduced with kind permission from the American Heart Journal.

the curves based on all other causes of death should also be shown, to confirm that the new intervention has not affected these (Figure 7.2).

7.4 Interpreting different types of phase III trials

The examples in Sections 7.1 to 7.3 were based on two-arm trials, which aimed to show whether one intervention was more effective than another (i.e. superiority). These approaches can be applied to other trial designs.

Crossover trials

Here, all subjects receive all the interventions. When the endpoint is 'taking measurements on people', each subject has two values (new intervention and control), and the difference is taken. The effect size is the mean of these differences over all subjects. Interpretation is the same as a mean difference from a two-arm trial (Section 7.2), and a 95% CI and p-value are calculated. If the trial endpoint is based on counting people, a 2×2 table can be constructed (Table 7.6). Patients who had an exacerbation on both interventions ($n = 8$) or

Table 7.6 Hypothetical results from a crossover trial comparing Treatment A with placebo in 100 patients with asthma. The outcome measure is the occurrence of an exacerbation or not.

		Placebo	
		Exacerbation	No exacerbation
Treatment A	Exacerbation	8	12
	No exacerbation	6	74

Table 7.7 Randomised double-blind factorial trial comparing folic acid and other multivitamins in preventing neural tube defect (NTD) pregnancies in 1195 women.[6]

Trial treatment		Number with an NTD pregnancy/ number in trial arm (%)	Relative risk (RR) calculation	
Folic acid	Other vitamins		Folic acid vs no folic acid	Other vitamins vs no other vitamins
Yes	No	2/298 (0.7)	$RR = \dfrac{(2+4)/(298+295)}{(13+8)/(300+302)}$	$RR = \dfrac{(4+8)/(295+302)}{(2+13)/(298+300)}$
Yes	Yes	4/295 (1.4)	$= 0.29$	$= 0.80$
No	No	13/300 (4.3)	95% CI $= 0.12$ to 0.71	95% CI $= 0.38$ to 1.70
No	Yes	8/302 (2.6)	p-value <0.0001	p-value $= 0.70$

had no exacerbations at all ($n = 74$) reveal nothing about whether Treatment A is better than placebo or not. However, the numbers on the diagonal are informative (6 vs 12); the **odds ratio** is 0.5 (6/12).[#] The odds of suffering an exacerbation on Treatment A is half that on placebo. Statistical methods are available to calculate a 95% CI and p-value for the odds ratio. Time-to-event endpoints are rarely, if ever, used in crossover trials.

The analysis of crossover trials can allow for a **period effect**; i.e. whether the effect size for Treatment B when preceded by A is different from Treatment A when preceded by B. Although the time interval between treatments should be long enough to minimise a **carryover effect** from one treatment to the next (see page 58), there are statistical methods that can allow for this.

Factorial trials

A factorial trial can efficiently compare two or more new interventions. Table 7.7 shows the results from a trial evaluating folic acid and other multivitamins in preventing neural-tube defect pregnancies.[6] A large (71%) risk reduction was associated with folic acid (relative risk 0.29), with a small p-value, but there was no evidence of an effect with other vitamins. The conclusion was to recommend folic acid only.

Factorial trials can also be used to detect an **interaction** between two interventions, i.e. if the effect size for one treatment depends on whether the subject has received the other treatment or not. In Figure 7.3, Treatment A increases the response rate by two percentage points (from 1 to 3% or 2 to 4%). Whether subjects also received Treatment B or not does not matter. There is no interaction. However, the effect of Treatment C depends on whether D was given, and vice versa: there is an interaction. Statistical methods can be used to investigate interactions (see Section 7.6), and provide p-values for them. When a clear interaction exists, the effect size for each treatment *combination* should be reported, as well as the main effect for each treatment.

[#] This has a different calculation to the odds ratio from a two-arm trial (Table 7.3).

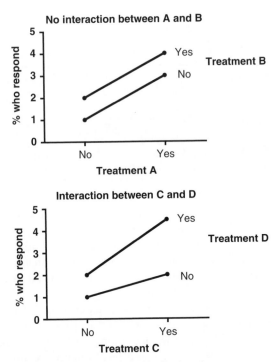

Figure 7.3 Illustration of an interaction between two treatments.

Equivalence and non-inferiority trials

For superiority trials one treatment is considered better than another when the CI for the effect size excludes the no-effect value, and the p-value is small (Box 7.6). For equivalence and non-inferiority trials the **maximum allowable**

Box 7.6 Interpreting different trials comparing interventions A and B

Objective:	Objective is met when:
Superiority (A is better than B)	95% confidence interval excludes the no-effect value
Equivalence (A is similar to B)	95% confidence interval includes the no-effect value and the interval is completely within the MAD range
Non-inferiority (A is not worse than B)	95% confidence interval does not cross one end of the MAD range (i.e. the end that indicates 'A' is worse)

MAD: maximum allowable difference

difference (MAD) is considered. This is a clinically important effect size, above which it is concluded that one intervention is better than the other (see page 67). When comparing two interventions which are expected to be similar, a p-value alone is of limited use. Although it needs to be ≥ 0.05, any trial with few subjects can produce large p-values, even when there is a real treatment effect. If the p-value is <0.05, it is likely that the two interventions have a different effect, and one might be chosen over the other.

Box 7.7 and Figure 7.4 show how to interpret data for equivalence or non-inferiority studies using 95% CIs. For equivalence trials, it is easiest to interpret results where the CI is completely within or completely outside of the MAD range. When the CI overlaps the MAD limit, it is not possible to reliably conclude whether the interventions have an equivalent effect or not. For non-inferiority studies, the new treatment is not considered worse than the control, if the CI does not cross the end of the MAD range associated with the new treatment being worse. Unless these trial types are large enough to produce precise estimates of treatment effect, CIs may be difficult to interpret.

Cluster randomised trial

The analyses described above apply to trials in which individual subjects are randomised to the trial interventions. In a cluster randomised trial, *groups* of people are randomised to each intervention (see page 61). A trial comparing two educational programmes could randomise schools to programme A or B. All children in the same school receive the same intervention. Variability exists between children in the same school, and between schools. Analysing the trial as if the children themselves were randomised, assumes independence in their responses. However, children within a school may be more similar than children between schools. Allowance should be made for this within-school variability (the **intra-class correlation**).

Suppose all children in a particular school have the same test score. Assessing more than one child from each school adds no information, and the number of independent observations would equal the number of schools. However, in reality, there would be variability within a school. By ignoring the within-school (intra-class) correlation, the p-value for an effect size could be smaller than it should be, producing a statistically significant result and an incorrect conclusion.[8,9] However, if the number of people within a cluster is small, the within-cluster variation will have a minimal effect, and the results of the trial should be similar to those obtained by assuming the data came from a standard trial where subjects themselves were randomised.

Repeated measures

When several measurements of the same endpoint are taken on each subject, they are likely to be correlated, and the effect size and p-value need to allow for this. A **repeated measures analysis of variance** or **covariance** can be performed. In the Atkins diet trial (Box 7.4), body weight was measured at three time points, and the data were analysed using this approach. The analysis

Box 7.7 Example of a phase III non-inferiority trial comparing two methods of delivering cognitive behavioural therapy to people with obsessive compulsive disorder (OCD)[7]

Location: 2 psychology outpatient departments in the UK

Subjects: 72 individuals aged ≥ 16 years with obsessive compulsive disorder

Design: Randomised controlled trial

Interventions: Cognitive behaviour therapy (10 weekly sessions) delivered either by telephone or face-to-face

Justification for trial: 'Face-to-face' therapy involves waiting lists and some people are unable to attend clinic appointments. Delivering therapy by telephone should increase access to treatment

Trial objective: 'Telephone' is not worse than 'face-to-face'

Main outcome measure: Score on the Yale Brown obsessive compulsive checklist (range 0 to 40, high score indicates more severe symptoms)

Maximum allowable difference (MAD): 5 units on the checklist (if the *true* mean difference is at least +5 units then 'telephone' is judged to be worse; if it is less than +5 then 'telephone' is not inferior)

72 individuals with OCD

36 telephone   36 face-to-face

Six months later
Yale Brown score
Mean (standard deviation)   14.2 (7.8)   13.3 (8.6)

Effect size: Adjusted mean difference +0.55, 95% CI (-3.15 to +4.26)

'Telephone' minus 'face-to-face'; adjusted for baseline score, hospital site and depression score

- The 95% CI for the *true* mean difference is between −3.15 and +4.26 units
- This is below +5 units, so 'telephone' is considered **not inferior**
- However, the 95% CI is completely within the MAD range of ±5 units, so it can also be concluded that the two interventions have an **equivalent** effect

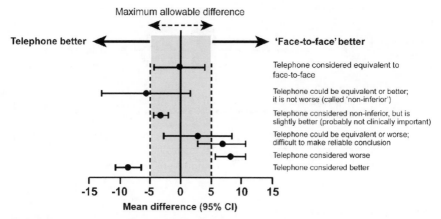

Figure 7.4 Illustration of interpreting effect sizes and confidence intervals from equivalence or non-inferiority trials using the example described in Box 7.7.
Objective: Comparing 'telephone' with 'face-to-face' delivery
Maximum allowable difference (MAD): 5 units on the Yale Brown obsessive compulsive checklist, indicated by the shaded region.
Mean difference = mean score using 'telephone' minus mean score using 'face-to-face' delivery.

could produce a single p-value for comparing the two diets, but also one for each time point (Table 7.4). **Mixed modelling** is another statistical method for this type of data. If multiple time points are analysed separately, the p-value for each should be inflated to allow for this.

There is sometimes a view that having a large trial can be avoided by measuring the same endpoint many times on fewer subjects. However, a study of 10 subjects, each with 10 measurements of the endpoint, is not the same as one measurement on 100 subjects. Although both produce 100 data values, there are still only 10 subjects in one study.

7.5 More on confidence intervals

The CI width depends on the standard error, which is derived from the trial size, and the number of events (when 'counting people' or using time-to-event endpoints), or the standard deviation (when 'taking measurements on people'). With few events, even a large trial could produce a large standard error. Generally, there is a relationship between study size and the strength of the conclusions that can be made (Figure 7.5).

Treatment effects are clearer, and the precision is higher, with large studies (Table 7.8). It is important, therefore, that the effect size used to calculate sample size is realistic enough to produce a big enough trial. Suppose the expected relative risk were 0.75, but the observed result was 0.85, with 95% CI 0.69 to 1.05. The upper limit is just above the no-effect value. The true effect size is probably closer to a 15% reduction in risk than a 25% reduction, but it requires a larger sample size to reliably show this, i.e. for the result to be statistically significant.

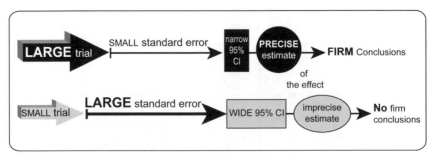

Figure 7.5 How study size affects conclusions.

7.6 More on p-values

The size of a p-value is influenced by the effect size and standard error. Large effect sizes or small standard errors produce small p-values. A small trial, or those with few events or large standard deviation, can each contribute to a large p-value (>0.05).

By convention, if the p-value is <0.05, the observed effect size is considered **statistically significant;** it is unlikely to have arisen by chance. If the p-value is ≥ 0.05, the effect size is **not statistically significant:** there is insufficient evidence of a true effect (Box 7.8). There is nothing very scientific about the cutoff of 0.05. It is generally accepted to indicate that a real effect is likely to exist because there is only a 1 in 20 likelihood that the results could have arisen by chance, assuming no true effect (i.e. a treatment effect could be falsely concluded 5% of the time). There is always some possibility, however small, that any observed effect size could be a chance finding, rather than reflect a real difference, but the smaller the p-value, the less likely that this is the case.

It is incorrect to conclude 'there is no effect' when the effect size is not statistically significant. It only means that there is insufficient evidence to claim an effect. P-values should not be reported as '<0.05', or '≥ 0.05' or 'Not statistically significant', because it is not possible to distinguish a p-value of 0.045 from <0.0001, or 0.06 from 0.57, yet they provide very different levels of evidence. If an effect size is not statistically significant, there are several reasons:

Table 7.8 Confidence intervals for trials with the same estimate of relative risk as in Box 7.1, but with different sample sizes.

	Risk in vaccine group	Risk in placebo group	Relative risk	Confidence interval
Trial 1/10 as big	4/90	8/90	0.50	0.16 to 1.60
Observed trial	41/927	80/911	0.50	0.35 to 0.72
Trial 10 times as big	410/9,270	800/9,100	0.50	0.44 to 0.56
Trial 100 times as big	4,100/92,700	8,000/91,000	0.50	0.48 to 0.52

Box 7.8 P-values

Definition: The probability that an effect as large as that observed, or more extreme, is due to chance *assuming* there really were no effect

All p-values are between 0 and 1

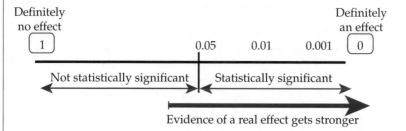

All p-values should be two-sided, except when one-sided tests are required because of the study design, such as in non-inferiority trials. In general, p-values larger than 0.01 should be reported to two decimal places, those between 0.01 and 0.001 to three decimal places, and those smaller than 0.001 should be reported as p < 0.001.

1. There really is no difference
2. There is a real difference, but by chance the sample of subjects did not show this
3. There is a real difference, but the trial had too few subjects, and therefore insufficient power, to detect it.

Large effect sizes can have p-values just above 0.05, such as 0.06. Although strictly not statistically significant, according to the 0.05 cut-off, a possible real treatment effect should not be dismissed. The trial was probably too small. Had it been larger, the p-value may have been smaller. Furthermore, a p-value of 0.048, while considered statistically significant, does not provide strong evidence of a treatment effect.

Calculating p-values

P-values come from performing a **statistical test**. The choice of test depends on the type of outcome measure. Some simple tests can be done by hand, but using a statistical software package avoids error, and they can cope easily with large datasets, providing all the information needed to interpret trial results, i.e. the effect size, 95% confidence interval and p-value. Box 7.9 shows some common statistical tests (details in the references on page 203). The multivariate (or multivariable) methods can be used to:

- Adjust for imbalances in baseline characteristics or other potential confounders (see page 88)

Box 7.9 Statistical methods that produce p-values according to type of endpoint (the multivariate and Cox's regression also provide effect sizes)

	Counting people (binary/ categorical data)	Taking measurements on people (continuous data)	Time-to-event data[4]
Two arm trial (unpaired data)	Chi-square test (or Fisher's exact test if the trial is small, <30)	Unpaired or two-sample t-test if the difference between the means is Normally distributed[1] Mann-Whitney U test if distribution of the difference is skewed[2]	Log rank test
Crossover or split-person trial (paired data)	McNemar's test	Paired t-test if the difference is Normally distributed Wilcoxon Matched pairs test if the distribution of the difference is skewed	Not applicable
Allow for other factors such as baseline imbalances	Multivariate logistic regression	Multivariate linear regression[3]	Cox's regression

1. With more than two trial arms the test is analysis of variance (ANOVA)
2. With more than two trial arms the test is Kruskal–Wallis ANOVA
3. Outcome measure should be approximately Normally distributed
4. If all subjects have the event of interest, tests for 'taking measurements on people' can be used

---

- Adjust for the stratification factors used in randomising subjects (see page 84)
- Investigate an interaction between a treatment and a prognostic factor (sub-group analyses, see page 119), or between two treatments (factorial trial).

Other methods, such as Bayesian statistics, attempt to incorporate prior evidence, but they are not commonly used to analyse clinical trials because of their complexity and the difficulty in determining how much importance should be given to the previous evidence.

Multiple endpoints

Some trials have several primary endpoints. Using the 0.05 p-value cut-off, an error rate of 5% is allowed, meaning that one spurious effect (false-positive result) is expected in every 20 comparisons. The more comparisons performed on the same data, the more likely that a spurious effect is found, i.e. an effect size with a p-value <0.05, but the effect was due to chance. When there are multiple primary outcome measures, p-values <0.05 might be adjusted using methods such as a Bonferroni correction. A p-value of 0.02 becomes 0.06 if there are three comparisons (0.02 × 3). However, this assumes the outcome measures are uncorrelated, which may not be true. Adjusting p-values in this way could inflate them too much, and a real treatment effect could be missed. A very small p-value (e.g. <0.001) is unlikely to be affected by several comparisons. It may be preferable to present the unadjusted p-values, with a suitable note of caution if they are just below 0.05, and 97.5% confidence intervals for say 2-3 comparisons, and 99% limits for ≥3, because they provide more conservative estimates of the range of the true effect.

7.7 Relationship between confidence intervals, the no-effect value and p-values

It can be inferred from the p-value whether the CI contains the no-effect value. The CI also indicates whether the effect size is statistically significant (Box 7.10). If the CI excludes the no-effect value, the result is statistically significant, otherwise, it is not statistically significant. This is because using a 95% CI and p-value cut-off of 5%, both allow an error rate of 5%.

Box 7.10 Relationship between confidence intervals and statistical significance

Effect size	No-effect value	95% confidence interval	p-value
• Relative risk • Odds ratio • Hazard ratio	1	includes 1	Effect size is not statistically significant (p-value ≥0.05)
		excludes 1	Effect size is statistically significant (p-value <0.05)
• Risk difference • % excess risk • % risk reduction • Difference between two means (or medians)	0	includes 0	Effect size is not statistically significant (p-value ≥0.05)
		excludes 0	Effect size is statistically significant (p-value <0.05)

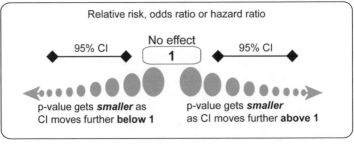

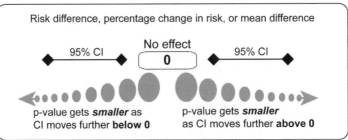

Figure 7.6 Relationship between confidence intervals and p-values. Sometimes it helps to consider how far the effect size is from the no-effect value in terms of number of standard errors. As this distance increases, the p-value gets smaller.

When the results are statistically significant, the size of the p-value can indicate how far the 95% CI is from the no-effect value (Figure 7.6). The smaller the p-value, the further away the CI. The results in Table 7.4 show this. The effect size at three months (−4.1 kg) has a small p-value (0.001) so the CI is far from the no-effect value. At six months, the p-value is larger (0.02) and the interval is closer to the no-effect value. A p-value of 0.05 indicates one of the limits is the no-effect value.

7.8 Intention-to-treat and per-protocol analyses

In Box 7.1, all randomised subjects received the allocated intervention (the flu vaccine). **Treatment compliance** was complete, i.e. 100%. In other studies, especially those that involve taking drugs or using medical devices at home, some people may not start treatment at all, and others will start, but stop before the protocol specifies they should. Also, the drug dose could be reduced, or subjects switch over to the other trial arm. These are all called **non-compliers**, and they often have different characteristics to compliers. There may be good reasons why subjects did not comply, such as intolerable side-effects. Any change from the protocol treatment schedule is a **protocol violation** or **deviation** ('violation' indicates one that could significantly affect the study design or results). A non-complier may be different from a subject who **withdraws** (page 118). The trial endpoint might be measurable on a non-complier, but not often for a withdrawal.

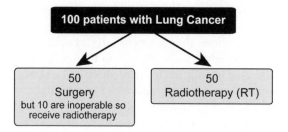

Possible ways of analysing this are:
(A) 40 surgery vs 60 RT (add the 10 inoperables to RT group)
(B) 40 surgery vs 50 RT (ignore the 10 inoperables)
(C) 40 surgery vs 40 RT (remove 10 from RT group)
(D) 50 surgery vs 50 RT (leave the 10 inoperables in the surgery group)

Figure 7.7 Hypothetical trial comparing two treatments in 100 patients with lung cancer, illustrating possible ways to deal with non-compliers to the allocated treatment. The main outcome could be survival after one year.

There are several ways of dealing with non-compliers in the analysis; see Figure 7.7. The 10 inoperable patients have more advanced disease, and therefore a poorer survival. Surgery would appear to have a better survival under options A and B, when there could be no real difference, because these patients are either ignored in the surgery group or, worse still, added to the radiotherapy group. In Option C, it is difficult to identify and remove 10 equivalent patients in the radiotherapy group to the 10 inoperable patients in the surgery group. Options A to C remove patients from the trial, or move them between arms, negating the balance achieved by the randomisation process, and possibly creating bias or confounding.

Option D is the most reasonable – called an **intention-to-treat analysis**. Subjects are analysed according to the arm to which they were randomised, regardless of whether they took the allocated intervention or not. This maintains the balance in baseline patient characteristics. The effect size reflects what could happen in practice, because not all people will take the intervention, or some may stop early because of side-effects. The analysis usually produces a conservative effect size because some people could have benefited from the new intervention had they taken it. However, the scientific advantage of having two balanced trial arms that are unaffected by bias or confounding, outweighs having an under-estimated effect size. All trials should be analysed in this way.

A **per-protocol analysis** only includes subjects who took their allocated treatment as specified in the trial protocol,[#] i.e. compliers (Option B in

---

[#] A non-complier can be defined in several ways in a particular trial. For example, it could be only those subjects who stopped treatment completely; those whose dose was reduced might still be regarded as compliers.

Figure 7.7). This is used for equivalence or non-inferiority trials. The endpoint is expected to be similar among non-compliers between the trial arms, so including them in an intention-to-treat analysis could make two interventions appear to have a more similar effect than they really do. A per-protocol analysis should be used in addition to an intention-to-treat analysis to confirm that the interventions have a comparable effect in compliers.

Examining the effect size only among those who did comply may also be useful when the proportion of compliers is clearly different between the trial arms (acknowledging that some balance in subject characteristics may be lost). Alternatively, a multi-variate method can produce an estimate of the effect size after allowing for level of compliance (Box 7.9). Again, these analyses could confirm consistency with the intention-to-treat analysis.

7.9 Randomised subjects who are ineligible and subject withdrawals

A randomised subject could be later found to be ineligible according to the inclusion and exclusion criteria; called a **protocol violation** or **deviation**. Small deviations should not matter, but large ones may. Suppose in a trial of newly diagnosed asthma patients, someone who has started the trial treatment is later found to not have asthma. He is, therefore, not expected to benefit from the new treatment, which would stop.

There are two options: include or exclude the subject from the analysis. Neither is perfect. The choice depends on the disease, the interventions being tested and how far the subject deviates from the eligibility criteria. When there are few ineligible subjects with significant protocol violations, they might be excluded. However, keeping them in would be consistent with an intention-to-treat analysis, because this is what would happen in practice. If there are many ineligible subjects, the reasons should be investigated. There may have been a problem with the trial design or recruitment. The number of ineligible subjects and the reasons should be recorded and reported.

Although trial subjects agree to participate until the end, some may withdraw early (**subject withdrawal, drop-out**, or **lost to follow up**), for example because of side-effects. When the endpoint is based on 'counting people', withdrawals can be included in the denominator of the risk in each arm. In the flu vaccine trial (Box 7.1), some subjects provided no blood sample, so it is not known whether they had serological flu at five months or not. There were 25 and 22 withdrawals in the vaccine and placebo groups respectively.[1] However, the risk of developing serological flu was based on the number randomised, and not 902 (927 – 25) and 889 (911 – 22). The endpoint could be thought of as '*known* serological flu'. With 'time-to-event' endpoints, subjects who withdraw are censored in the analysis at the time they were last seen.

In both cases, all subjects can be included in an intention-to-treat analysis, though some statistical power might be reduced because the number of events is less than the number originally expected. A loss of power could be avoided by inflating the target sample size to allow for possible withdrawals.

However, when 'taking measurements on people', it is difficult to include withdrawals since there is no value to use in calculating the mean (or median). Such subjects are often excluded from the analysis, though statistical methods, called **imputation**, can attempt to estimate the missing values.

When there are relatively few withdrawals and the number is similar between the trial arms, the results are unlikely to be materially affected if such patients are excluded. Attempts should be made to try to ensure that the number of patient withdrawals is kept to a minimum, but if these do occur, they should be recorded and mentioned in the final report.

7.10 Sub-group analyses

The effect size is often examined to see if it differs between sub-groups of subjects (e.g. by gender). The ultimate purpose of this should be clear. If the benefit is greater in a certain group of subjects than another, but there is still a clear benefit in both groups, all future subjects would still be offered the new treatment; the sub-group analysis simply provides additional information about the treatment. A problem arises when a sub-group analysis is used to determine who will and will not receive the new treatment. There needs to be very clear and convincing data on this, in order to avoid withholding an effective therapy from future individuals.

Sub-group analyses should be specified at the start of the trial in the protocol, or performed when there is good scientific justification. Otherwise, they could look like a 'fishing expedition'. This is particularly so when no overall treatment effect is found, and sub-groups are examined in the hope of finding an effect. Alternatively, the effect of a new intervention in a particular sub-group could, by chance, appear larger than it really is. If there is prior evidence that a treatment effect is influenced by important prognostic factors, the sample size could be increased to allow sufficient statistical power to examine this reliably.

Sub-group analyses are usually presented as a **forest plot** (Figure 7.8). For example, the relative risks and 95% CIs are 0.36 (0.13 to 0.97) among males and 0.68 (0.33 to 1.43) among females. It is incorrect to conclude that the vaccine was effective in males, but not in females because one CI excludes the no-effect value, and the other includes it.[10] The point estimates for both males and females indicate a benefit, but the wide CIs come from having a smaller sample size in each sub-group. What matters is whether the CIs do not overlap, or they exclude the overall effect size. In Figure 7.8, no factor does this. Another approach is to perform a multi-variate statistical analysis (Box 7.9) and obtain a p-value for an **interaction** or **heterogeneity test**.

There are several issues to consider. First, dividing the data into smaller groups of subjects produces wider 95% CIs making it more difficult to find statistically significant results. Second, if very different effect sizes are found between the sub-groups, some plausible explanation is expected, which may be difficult. Third, the more sub-group analyses performed, the more likely that a spurious treatment effect is found. An example is shown in Table 7.9.[11]

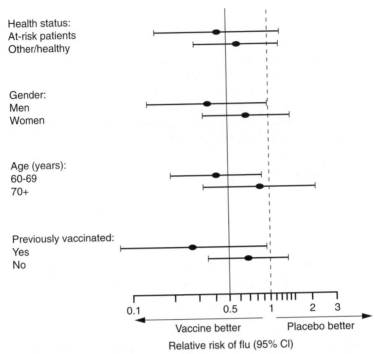

Figure 7.8 Forest plot showing the results of sub-group analyses in the flu vaccine trial (Box 7.1), based on clinician-diagnosed flu five months after vaccination. The figure shows the effect size, i.e. relative risk, in different groups of trial subjects. The solid vertical line is the relative risk among all subjects (0.50), and the dashed line is the no-effect value.

Table 7.9 Trial of aspirin versus placebo in treating 17,000 patients with suspected acute myocardial infarction.[11]

| Astrological sign | % with vascular death after 1 month* | | Relative risk (95% confidence interval) | p-value |
	Aspirin N = 8553	Placebo N = 8610		
Libra or Gemini	11.1%	10.2%	1.09 (0.88 – 1.35)	0.50
All other signs	9.0%	12.1%	0.74 (0.68 – 0.82)	<0.0001
All patients	9.4%	11.8%	0.80 (0.73 – 0.87)	<0.0001

*there were 1820 deaths in total

The number of patients in each group and the confidence intervals were estimated from data given in the reference.[11]

Aspirin appears to be only effective in people who were not Libra or Gemini, but there is no biological plausibility for this. Large trials can produce spurious subgroup results that are precise, with statistically significant interactions. Adding the caveat that any such sub-group analysis should be viewed with caution may not avoid them being misinterpreted.

Consideration should be given to whether sub-group analyses are a sensible approach, and to the possibility of finding false-positive effects. It may be preferable not to present any, or they should be used to generate hypotheses for further studies.

7.11 Safety, toxicity or adverse events

Table 7.10 shows selected side-effects from a trial of patients with osteoarthritis or rheumatoid arthritis.[12] Effect sizes and 95% CIs could be presented for each row, but the table could look unwieldy. Instead, summary measures are presented for groups of side-effects. The sum of the numbers with gastrointestinal effects in the NSAID group (640 + 522 + 392 + 370 + 234) is 2158, greater than the total of 1465. This is because patients can have more than one type of event, so appear in more than one row. It should be made clear whether the number of events or number of patients with an event is reported. Where people can suffer several (perhaps related) side-effects, it is usually preferable

Table 7.10 The number of patients with specified side-effects from a randomised trial comparing Celecoxib (a COX 2-specific inhibitor) and nonsteroidal anti-inflammatory drugs (NSAIDs) for treating osteoarthritis and rheumatoid arthritis.[12]

Side-effects after six months of treatment	NSAID N = 3981	Celecoxib N = 3987
	n (%)	n (%)
Gastrointestinal		
Dyspepsia	640 (16.1)	575 (14.4)
Abdominal pain	522 (13.1)	387 (9.7)
Diarrhoea	392 (9.8)	373 (9.4)
Nausea	370 (9.3)	277 (6.9)
Constipation	234 (5.9)	68 (1.7)
Any (each patient counted once)	1465 (36.8)	1250 (31.4)
Risk difference % & 95% confidence interval*	+5.4 (+3.4 to +7.5) p-value < 0.0001	
Cardiovascular		
Stroke	10 (0.3)	5 (0.1)
Myocardial infarction	11 (0.3)	10 (0.3)
Angina	22 (0.6)	24 (0.6)
Any (each patient counted once)	39 (1.0)	37 (0.9)
Risk difference % & 95% confidence interval*	+0.05 (−0.4 to +0.5) p-value = 0.81	

*estimated using the reported results

to report the number of affected subjects rather than the number of events, because the extent of harm in one trial arm could be over-estimated. When a particular side-effect is recorded on several occasions a common approach is to report the most severe grade for each subject.

In Table 7.10, the risk of suffering a gastrointestinal toxicity was greater in the NSAID group than in the Celecoxib group (36.8 vs 31.4%). The relative risk was 1.17 (36.8 ÷ 31.4%), with 95% CI 1.10 to 1.25. NSAIDs increased the risk of having a gastrointestinal side-effect by 17%. The absolute risk difference (+5.4%) perhaps better indicates the extent of harm, because it gives the number of affected individuals. In 100 patients given NSAIDs an *extra* 5.4 are expected to have a gastrointestinal side-effect, compared with 100 given Celecoxib. The **number needed to harm (NNH)** is 18 (100/5.4), similar in principle to number needed to treat (Box 7.2). For every 18 patients given NSAIDs, one extra patient with a gastrointestinal side-effect is expected that is attributable to NSAIDs, compared to the Celecoxib group.

The results in Table 7.10 are for a treatment period of six months, but it is sometimes important to detect late effects.

7.12 Interim analyses and stopping trials early

Interim analyses involve examining the data when subjects are still being recruited or sometimes treated. They could be used to change the trial design, or decide whether the trial should continue or stop early.

Revising the sample size may be necessary when the early analysis indicates that the effect size used in the sample-size calculation was too large, or there are fewer events than expected. This could be due to having narrow eligibility criteria, or improvements in the standard of care. Increasing the sample size or length of follow up, should increase the number of events. Sample size should not be reduced when the effect size used in the sample-size calculation is later considered too small, unless there is clear and convincing evidence for this.

A trial may stop early for several reasons:
- *Poor recruitment* – the trial is highly unlikely to finish in a reasonable time-frame
- *New evidence* – information becomes available, perhaps from another trial, which makes recruitment to one or more arms of the current trial unethical or unacceptable
- *Harm* – the new intervention is clearly more harmful than the control. It is almost always appropriate to consider stopping early when this occurs
- *Superiority* – the new treatment is judged with sufficient certainly to be more beneficial than the control
- *Futility* – it is judged that there is unlikely to be a clinically important treatment effect if the trial continued to the end. Alternatively, if the new intervention has more side-effects or is more expensive, the true effect size is unlikely to be large enough to justify its use.

The number and timing of the interim analyses can depend on the interventions being tested, but one or two, say after half or a third/two thirds of subjects have been recruited, often seems appropriate. There could be more analyses, particularly early on, if the focus is on safety.

Safety is assessed by determining whether adverse events are likely to be caused by the trial treatment, and examining their severity and frequency, and whether they are easily treated. This is often separate from harm that is directly associated with the efficacy outcome measure (see page 181).

Stopping early for superiority may be justified when there is a large effect size and a narrow 95% CI. A **stopping rule** involves pre-specifying a p-value cut-off at each interim analysis, below which the recommendation is to stop the trial. The p-value used for the final analysis may then be reduced. Smaller p-values could be specified at earlier analyses because stronger evidence is required when there are relatively few subjects.[13] For example, with two interim analyses, the first p-value could be <0.0005, and the second <0.014. To claim statistical significance in the final analysis, the p-value would need to be <0.045.[#] The overall p-value, allowing for three analyses, is about 5%. Alternatively, a stringent stopping rule is to specify that any interim p-value must be <0.001 (referred to as the Peto–Haybittle rule). The cut-off for the final analysis p-value could still be 0.05.[#] Sample size can be increased to allow for interim analyses.

Stopping early for futility can be difficult. Current trial data is used to predict the future effect size if the trial continued. Complex statistical methods can estimate the probability of getting the expected effect size in the future given the data now, but they are based on several assumptions. Examining the 95% CI gives a simple estimate of the future true effect size. If it completely excludes a clinically important difference, the intervention is unlikely to be effective. For example, finding a lower confidence limit of 0.96 when the expected relative risk is 0.75.

Several considerations arise when interpreting interim analyses of efficacy.[14] First, a statistically significant effect could be found, when there really is no effect, if many analyses are performed. This is minimised by having a stringent stopping rule. Second, the analyses could be based on a sample size that would not persuade health professionals to change practice. An interim analysis of 10,000 subjects, out of a target of 20,000, is probably sufficiently large, particularly if there are many events. However, halfway through a two-arm trial with a target of 500 subjects represents only 125 in each arm. The effect size might be statistically significant, but with a wide CI, which would not be convincing enough to change practice. (See the results for 'new

---

[#] It is not 5% because some of the allowed 5% error rate has been 'used up' at early analyses, called alpha spending (the error rate can be notated by α). In the Peto–Haybittle rule, very little of the 5% has been spent early on, so the final p-value can still be compared against 0.05.

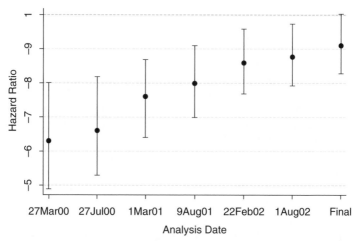

Figure 7.9 Several interim analyses in a trial comparing Candesartan with placebo, and the effect on cardiovascular (CV) death.[5] Reproduced with kind permission from the American Heart Journal.

tumour' in Table 7.5; an apparently large effect, but based on few events.) Third, treatment effects could be greater earlier on. In Figure 7.9,[5] the March 2000 analysis showed a large effect size with a p-value of 0.0006. However, at the end of the trial, the effect was smaller and only close to statistically significance (p = 0.055). Large early treatment effects could be 'too good to be true'.

All the relevant evidence needs to be considered before stopping early, not just statistical stopping rules and p-values. Other considerations include the success of recruitment, any safety issues, whether there is sufficient evidence to change practice or if a clinically important effect is highly unlikely if the trial continued. When a trial is stopped too early, the data might not be reliable enough to persuade the regulatory authority to grant a marketing licence for a new therapy, or an effective treatment may not be found because the early analysis suggested futility.

7.13 Clinical versus statistical significance: more on interpreting results

P-values are often used to drive the interpretation of clinical trial data, and too much emphasis is placed on whether it crosses the conventional cut-off of 0.05, i.e. **statistical significance**. P-values only provide an indication of whether the observed effect size could be due to chance, so they should be used as a *guide* to interpreting data. There should be more focus on interpreting the observed effect size and CIs, i.e. **clinical significance**.

Consider hypothetical results of trials evaluating four new diets (Box 7.11). When trials are large, precise estimates of the effect size are obtained so it is clear whether the new intervention is likely to be clinically worthwhile (Diet

---

Box 7.11 Hypothetical clinical trials of four new diets for weight loss. Effect size is the mean difference in weight (intervention arm minus control arm)

		Clinical significance?	
		Yes	No
Statistical significance?	Yes	Diet A $N = 1,000$ Mean difference −7.0 kg 95% CI −7.6 to −6.4 kg p-value <0.0001 *Big study* *Big effect*	Diet B $N = 2,000$ Mean difference −0.5 kg 95% CI −0.9 to −0.1 kg p-value = 0.025 *Big study* *Small effect*
	No	Diet C $N = 36$ Mean difference −3.0 kg 95% CI −6.3 to +0.3 kg P-value = 0.07 *Study not big enough* *Probably a real & moderate effect,* *but insufficient results to draw a* *reliable conclusion*	Diet D $N = 400$ Mean difference −0.2 kg 95% CI −1.2 to +0.8 kg P-value = 0.69 *Study probably big enough* *Probably small effect*

'N' is the total number of subjects in a two-arm trial

A in Box 7.11) or not (Diet D). A statistically significant result could be found in large studies when the effect is small and clinically unimportant (Diet B).

Perhaps the most difficult results to interpret occur when the p-value is just above 0.05, but the effect size looks large (Diet C). Although the CI includes the no-effect value, most of the range is below zero. The data must be interpreted carefully. 'There is no effect' should not be concluded, because the true mean difference could be as large as 6 kg. It is better to say 'there is some evidence of an effect, but the result has just missed statistical significance', or 'there is a suggestion of an effect'. Using language like this does not dismiss outright what could be a real effect, but it also makes no undue claims about efficacy.

7.14 Summary

- A summary effect size can be obtained for any comparison of two interventions

- The type of effect size and how it is analysed depends on the type of outcome measure – counting people, taking measurements or time-to-event data:
  - Counting people: risk difference, relative risk, odds ratio
  - Taking measurements on people: difference between two means or medians
  - Time-to-event: hazard ratio, difference between two survival or event rates
- Confidence intervals and p-values must be calculated for any effect size, to fully interpret the data
- Design considerations help when interpreting results; two-arm, crossover and factorial trials; repeated measures
- Sub-group analyses should be justified and specified at the start of the trial, and interpreted carefully
- Large trials, with many events, should produce the clearest results and conclusions.

References

1. Govaert TME, Thijs CTMCN, Masurel N et al. The efficacy of influenza vaccination in elderly individuals. *JAMA* 1994; **272**(21): 1661–1665.
2. Foster GD, Wyatt HR, Hill JO et al. A randomized trial of a low carbohydrate diet for obesity. *N Engl J Med* 2003; **348**:2082–2090.
3. Vickers AJ, Altman DG. Analysing controlled trials with baseline and follow-up measurements. *BMJ* 2001; **323**:1123–1124.
4. Romond EH, Perez EA, Bryant J et al. Trastuzumab plus Adjuvant Chemotherapy for Operable HER2-Positive Breast Cancer. *N Eng J Med* 2005; **353**:1673–1684.
5. Pocock S, Wang D, Wilhelmsen L, Hennekens C. The data monitoring experience in the Candesartan in Heart Failure Assessment of Reduction in Mortality and morbidity (CHARM) program. *Am Heart J* 2005; **149**:939–943.
6. MRC Vitamin Study Research Group. Prevention of neural tube defects: results of the MRC vitamin study. *The Lancet* 1991; **338**:132–137.
7. Lovell K, Cox D, Haddock G et al. Telephone administered cognitive behaviour therapy for treatment of obsessive compulsive disorder: randomised controlled non-inferiority trial. *BMJ* 2006; **333**:883–887.
8. Kerry SM, Bland JM. Analysis of a trial randomised in clusters. *BMJ* 1998; **316**:54.
9. Bland JM, Kerry SM. The intracluster correlation coefficient in cluster randomisation. *BMJ* 1998; **316**:1455–1460.
10. Cuzick J. Forest plots and the interpretation of subgroups. *The Lancet* 2005; **365**:1308.
11. Collins R, MacMahon S. Reliable assessment of the effects of treatment on mortality and major morbidity, I: clinical trials. *The Lancet* 2001; **357**:373–380.
12. Silverstein FE, Faich G, Goldstein JL et al. Gastrointestinal toxicity with Celecoxib vs nonsteroidal anti-inflammatory drugs for osteoarthritis and rheumatoid arthritis. The CLASS Study: a randomised controlled trial. *JAMA* 2000; **284**:1247–1255.
13. O'Brien PC, Fleming TR. A multiple testing procedure for clinical trials. *Biometrics* 1979; **35**:549–556.
14. Pocock SJ. When to stop a clinical trial. *BMJ* 1992; **305**:235–240.

Appendix: Further introduction to p-values

Suppose a coin is to be thrown 10 times. If a Heads appears after one throw, there is no reason to think there is anything unusual about the coin. If two Heads are seen in a row, this is also not surprising. If, however, five Heads are seen in a row, suspicions are aroused, and after 10 Heads, there is a readiness to believe that something is wrong with the coin. But on what evidence are the suspicions based? If the coin were fair, the chance of getting Heads (or Tails) is 0.5. Therefore, among 10 throws of the coin about five Heads and five Tails are expected. What we are doing mentally after each successive result is considering whether what is seen is consistent with the *assumption* that the coin is fair. We might never be able to determine if the coin is fair or not with complete certainty. However, it is the assumption of fairness (i.e. probability of 0.5 of seeing Heads) that we use to judge the coin as it is thrown.

The probability of throwing five Heads in a row *if the coin were fair* is 0.03 (0.5^5), i.e. 3 in 100. This means that if there were five throws of the coin, and this was repeated 100 times, five Heads in a row is expected to occur in three out of the 100 sets, just by chance. Similarly, the probability of seeing 10 Heads in a row due to chance is 0.001 (0.5^{10}), i.e. in 1,000 sets each consisting of 10 throws, 10 consecutive Heads could be seen among one set. So it is not impossible to get 10 Heads in a row with a fair coin – it is just very unlikely. The table below shows the probability of getting various combinations of Heads and Tails in 10 throws of the coin. Each number in the third column is the p-value associated with the particular result of the coin thrown 10 times.

Number of Heads	Number of Tails	Probability of this occurring if the coin were fair*
0	10	0.0010
1	9	0.0097
2	8	0.0440
3	7	0.1172
4	6	0.2051
5	5	0.2460
6	4	0.2051
7	3	0.1172
8	2	0.0440
9	1	0.0097
10	0	0.0010
Total		1.0000

*i.e. the chance of a Heads is 0.5

Suppose there were one Heads and nine Tails. We would not necessarily be interested only in this particular combination but also one that is more extreme, i.e. 0 Heads and 10 Tails. The probability of this is $0.0097 + 0.001 = 0.0107$. This is referred to as a **one-tailed p-value**. However, getting one Heads and nine Tails is as suspicious as nine Heads and one Tails. What is needed is a p-value for the one vs nine or more extreme, and in either direction. The probability of this is $0.0097 + 0.001 + 0.0097 + 0.001 = 0.021$. This is a **two-tailed p-value**.

The same principles apply to interpreting clinical trial results. In the flu vaccine trial (Box 7.1), the risk difference is -4.4%. To judge whether an effect at least as large as this could be due to chance, the calculation of the p-value *assumes* that the true risk difference is zero (i.e. there is no effect). The p-value of <0.001 is associated with an effect as large as 4.4% or more extreme in either direction (i.e. $\leq -4.4\%$ or $\geq +4.4\%$), which allows for the vaccine to be better or worse than placebo. Again, it is not impossible for a trial to produce a treatment effect this large if there really were no effect, but the p-value here tells us that this is extremely unlikely.

Observed result	We assume	P-value
Coin		
One Heads vs nine Tails	Probability of Heads is 0.5 and Observed result could be more extreme in either direction	0.021
Flu vaccine trial		
Risk difference -4.4%	No effect (true risk difference $= 0$) and Observed result could be more extreme in either direction	<0.001

CHAPTER 8

Systematic reviews and meta-analyses

Previous chapters presented key features of the design, analysis and interpretation of a single clinical trial. When there are several similar trials on the same subject, it is possible to review the accumulation of evidence, and provide a clearer view on the effectiveness of a particular intervention.

Large trials usually provide robust results, allowing unambiguous conclusions to be made. In small trials, it can be difficult to detect a treatment effect, if one exists, and statistical significance is often not achieved (the p-value is ≥ 0.05). This means that a real effect could be missed, and there is uncertainty over whether the observed result is real or due to chance.

The limitations of small trials could be largely overcome by combining them in a single analysis. This is the main purpose of a systematic review and meta-analysis. Systematic reviews are different from review articles, which may be presented as narratives based on selected papers, and may therefore reflect the personal professional interests of the author: there could be a bias towards the positive (or negative) studies. Such reviews tend to describe the features of each paper without trying to combine the results. The assessment of several trials together needs to be done in a **systematic** and unbiased way.

8.1 The need for systematic reviews of clinical trials

Systematic reviews tend to be conducted on randomised phase II or III trials, rather than single-arm trials, and there are three broad functions:

- *To confirm existing practice but provide a more precise estimate of the treatment effect.* By considering several trials together, the results are combined to give a single estimate of the effect size. The standard error of the pooled effect size is usually smaller than for any individual trial. As a consequence, the 95% confidence interval will be the narrowest, i.e. the effect size will have greater precision, and the result is more likely to be statistically significant. By having a larger number of subjects in the analysis, it is also possible to detect smaller treatment effects than those normally found in individual trials. Also, sub-group analyses are based on more patients than in any individual trial, and so have greater statistical power, though spurious effects could still be found by chance if many sub-groups are examined (see page 119).

A concise guide to clinical trials, First edition. By A. Hackshaw. Published 2009 by Blackwell Publishing, ISBN: 978-1-4051-6774-1.

- *To change existing practice*. Some systematic reviews have changed health practice. Occasionally, they have led to a new intervention being adopted into practice, but usually they have resulted in an existing treatment becoming more commonly used. Examples are tamoxifen and breast cancer, streptokinase and acute myocardial infarction, and aspirin and stroke. Such reviews are often used to develop national guidelines for defining standard practice.
- *To determine whether new trials are needed*. When there is uncertainty over the effectiveness of an intervention, a systematic review of the literature can help decide whether a new trial is needed. In this situation, there are usually only a few small published trials. The purpose is to determine whether these trials taken together would provide sufficient evidence of the treatment effect, because if they do not, having a large new trial is justified.

8.2 What is a systematic review?

Systematic reviews apply a formal methodological approach to obtaining, analysing and interpreting all the available reports on a particular topic. In an era of evidence-based health, where health professionals are encouraged to identify sources of evidence for their work, and to keep abreast of new developments, systematic reviews are valuable summaries of the evidence. A review is a research project in its own right and, depending on the number of published reports to be considered, can be a lengthy undertaking. The review is only as good as the studies on which it is based. If an area has been investigated mainly using small, poorly designed trials, a review of these may not be a substitute for a single large well-designed trial.

The systematic review process is given in Box 8.1. The summary data (i.e. effect sizes) can be extracted from the published papers. Alternatively, the raw data is requested from the authors, called an **individual patient data (IPD) meta-analysis**, and once it is sent to a central depository, there is essentially a single large data set with a variable that identifies each original trial. Such analyses can produce a more precise estimate of the combined effect size than using summary data, and more reliable sub-group analyses.

Systematic reviews can take from a few weeks up to two or more years, depending on how many trials there are and the type of meta-analysis. Those based on IPD can be lengthy and require dedicated resources because the raw data needs to be collected, collated and checked before conducting the statistical analyses and writing the report.

8.3 Sources of published systematic reviews

The Cochrane Collaboration is a well-known collection of systematic reviews. It covers a wide range of clinical disciplines, and the reviews are available on the Internet. They are limited to clinical trials of detection, prevention or treatment. There are about 40 established Collaborative Review Groups, within

---

Box 8.1 Stages of a systematic review

1. Define the research question, and identify the appropriate outcome measures
2. Specify a list of criteria for including and excluding studies
3. Undertake a literature search (using medical databases, for example, PubMed, Medline and Embase) and after reading the abstracts identify articles that might be appropriate
4. Obtain the full papers identified from the literature search. The reference lists of these papers could be used to identify additional papers not found in the electronic search
5. Critically appraise each report and extract specific relevant information. Clearly defined outcome measures are essential
6. Perform a **meta-analysis** which involves combining the quantitative results from the individual studies into a single estimate
7. Interpret and summarise the findings.

---

which systematic reviews are prepared to a similar standard, and sometimes updated regularly:

- Cochrane Collaboration (`http://www.cochrane.org`)
- The Cochrane Library (`http://www3.interscience.wiley.com/cgi-bin/mrwhome/106568753/HOME`)

Systematic reviews and meta-analyses can also be found in electronic databases of clinical and psychology journals:

- Medline (`http://medline.cos.com/`)
- Embase (`http://www.embase.com/`)
- PubMed (`http://www.ncbi.nlm.nih.gov/entrez/query.fcgi`)

These databases contain abstracts of most scientific published articles, and they have keyword search facilities. Systematic review articles should be categorised as such, but using keywords such as 'systematic review' or 'meta analysis' in a search should ensure that all these articles are retrieved.

National governmental organisations, which often fund external systematic reviews or conduct them internally, may also list completed reviews on their website. In the UK, for example these include:

- The UK Health Technology Assessment (`http://www.ncchta.org/`)
- National Institute for Health and Clinical Excellence, NICE (`http://www.nice.org.uk/`)
- The Centre for Reviews and Dissemination (CRD) in York (`http://www.york.ac.uk/inst/crd/`)

8.4 Interpreting systematic reviews

Systematic reviews of clinical trials usually focus on those that compare two or more groups of people, so that an effect size is available, for example, relative risk, risk difference, hazard ratio, or mean difference. It is worth clarifying the following points:

- What is the aim of the review? This is often similar to the main objective of a single trial.
- How was the review conducted?
- What are the main outcome measures?
- What are the main results? The pooled effect size and corresponding confidence interval and p-value can be interpreted as described in Chapter 7.

Meta-analysis

The main stage of a systematic review is combining the effect sizes into a single estimate using a statistical technique called **meta-analysis**. If a simple average of the effect size were taken, small and large studies would have the same influence in the analysis, but there needs to be some way of taking into account that one trial may be based on 100 people and another on 1,000 (this is described below).

Figure 8.1 is a typical meta-analysis plot (a **forest plot**), associated with a review of nicotine replacement therapy (NRT). It shows the individual results from 13 randomised trials of self-referred smokers, in which subjects were randomised to receive either 2 mg nicotine chewing gum or control (such as placebo gum). The main outcome measure is the proportion of smokers who had stopped smoking one year after starting treatment, and the effect size is

Review: The effect of nicotine replacement therapy on smoking cessation
Comparison: 01 2mg nicotine chewing gum versus control
Outcome: 01 The proportion of smokers who had stopped smoking at one year

Sudy or sub-category	2mg nicotine gum n/N	Control n/N	RR (fixed) 95% CI	Weight %	RR (fixed) 95% CI
Areechon 1988	56/99	37/101		12.34	1.54 [1.13, 2.10]
Clavel 1985	24/205	6/222		1.94	4.33 [1.81,10.38]
Fagerstrom 1982	30/50	22/50		7.41	4.36 [0.93, 2.01]
Fee 1982	23/180	15/172		5.17	1.47 [0.79, 2.71]
Hall 1987	30/71	14/68		4.82	2.05 [1.20, 3.52]
Hjalmarson 1984	29/106	16/100		5.55	1.71 [0.99, 2.95]
Hughes 1990	8/20	7/39		1.60	2.23 [0.94, 5.26]
Jarvik 1984	7/25	4/23		1.40	1.61 [0.54, 4.79]
Jarvis 1982	27/58	12/58		4.04	2.25 [1.27, 4.00]
Killen1984	11/22	6/20		2.12	1.67 [0.76, 3.67]
Killen 1990	127/600	106/618		35.17	1.23 [0.98, 1.56]
Malcolm 1980	17/73	5/63		1.81	2.93 [1.15, 7.50]
Pirie 1992	75/206	50/211		16.64	1.54 [1.14, 2.08]
Total (95% CI)	1715	1745		100.00	1.57 [1.39, 1.78]

Total events: 464 (2mg nicotine gum), 300 (Control)
Test for heterogeneity: Chi² = 14.83, df = 12 (P = 0.25), I² = 19.1%
Test for overall effect: Z = 7.11 (P < 0.00001)

```
        0.1 0.2   0.5  1   2    5   10
      Favours control   Favours 2mg gum
```

Figure 8.1 Example of a forest plot from a meta-analysis; randomised trials evaluating nicotine replacement therapy (2 mg nicotine chewing gum) and the effect on smoking cessation rates.[1] The figure was obtained using RevMan.[3] RR: relative risk; CI: confidence interval; n: number of events, i.e. number of people who quit smoking; N: number randomised in each trial arm. The no-effect value is 1.0. If the 95% CI excludes one, the result is statistically significant.

the relative risk (the ratio of these proportions). The studies are listed in alphabetical order according to the first author, but they could also be ordered by year of publication or magnitude of the effect size. Forest plots can be derived for any type of effect size.

An important observation is that all trials have a relative risk greater than the no-effect value: the proportion of smokers who quit was always higher in the NRT group. If there really were no association between NRT and quit rate, some trials should have a relative risk below one. Although several trials had statistically significant results (e.g. Areechon 1988 and Clavel 1985), others did not. Even the largest trial by Killen (1990) just missed statistical significance; lower confidence limit was 0.98. Because of this, a meta-analysis of all the results seems appropriate in order to provide a clearer conclusion on the effect of NRT.

Large trials usually have small standard errors, which produces estimates of the true effect size that are more precise than those from trials with large standard errors. The **weight** given to each trial is calculated from the **standard error** of the relative risk, on a log scale (Box 8.2). In Figure 8.1, each weight is expressed as a percentage of the sum of all the weights across trials, allowing a comparison of the relative contribution that each trial makes to the analysis.

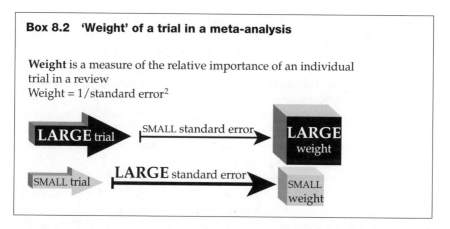

Box 8.2 'Weight' of a trial in a meta-analysis

Weight is a measure of the relative importance of an individual trial in a review

Weight $= 1/$standard error^2

Trials with small standard errors have narrow confidence intervals and therefore larger weights. For example, the large trial by Killen (1990) in Figure 8.1 has 35.17% of all the relative weights. Trials with large standard errors have wider confidence intervals (e.g. Jarvik 1984) and a smaller weight (1.4%). It should be noted that the trial by Clavel (1985) was the second largest, but the standard error was large because the number of events (i.e. smokers who quit) was small. The size of the trial and the number of events influences the magnitude of the standard error. Forest plots usually make the size of the central square for each trial proportional to the weight, making trials with small standard errors more prominent to the eye.

The statistical techniques used in a meta-analysis allow for the weight of each trial when combining the effect sizes (the simplest method is shown in

Box 8.3). The combined estimate of the relative risk of NRT compared with control is shown as the large diamond in the row labelled 'Total' in Figure 8.1. It is 1.57, with a 95% CI of 1.39 to 1.78 (the ends of the diamond). Smokers given 2 mg nicotine chewing gum were 57% more likely to quit at one year than smokers in the control group, and the true excess risk is likely to lie between 39% and 78%. This range is narrower than any trial on its own. The p-value associated with the combined estimate is very small, $p < 0.00001$ (see 'Test for overall effect'), which is highly statistically significant: the observed effect is unlikely to be due to chance.

Box 8.3   Estimating the combined effect size (fixed effects model)

$$\text{Combined effect size} = \frac{\text{sum of (effect size} \times \text{weight for each trial)}}{\text{sum of all the weights}}$$

The effect size could be a mean difference, absolute risk difference, relative risk or hazard ratio (the latter two are used on a $\log_e$ scale, and the result is anti-logged).

Heterogeneity

No two trials are identical in design and conduct, so it is necessary to consider whether the observed effect sizes materially differ from each other, i.e. whether there is **heterogeneity**, and if it is appropriate to combine the results into a single estimate. Figure 8.2 illustrates this using four hypothetical studies. Studies 1 to 3 appear similar (no heterogeneity), but Study 4 clearly looks different from the other three (evidence of heterogeneity). Statistical tests can determine whether significant heterogeneity is present. When it is, statistical methods can combine the effect sizes to allow for it.[2]

In Figure 8.1, a **test for heterogeneity** (shown in the bottom left-hand corner) produced a p-value of 0.25, suggesting that the relative risk estimates do not differ substantially from each other. Here, an appropriate method to combine the results is a 'fixed effects model', indicated by the word 'fixed' at the top right-hand side. If there is significant heterogeneity (i.e. the p-value for the test is <0.05), a 'random effects model' may be more appropriate, because this method takes into account variability between studies. The word 'fixed' would be replaced with 'random'. The two methods tend to produce similar effect sizes and CIs when there is little or no heterogeneity. When there is significant heterogeneity, the pooled effect sizes are usually similar but the 'random effects' approach produces wider confidence intervals to allow for the between-trial variability; there is more uncertainty over the size of the true effect given the greater variability. In the example, the combined relative risks and 95% CIs are 1.57 (1.39 to 1.78) and 1.61 (1.38 to 1.86) using the fixed and random models respectively.

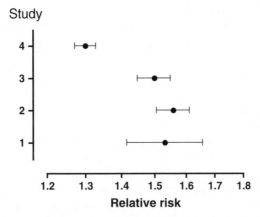

Figure 8.2 Illustration of heterogeneity among four hypothetical trials. The results from Trials 1 to 3 are similar, but the result from Trial 4 is clearly different.

The standard test for heterogeneity is not very powerful in detecting differences between trials when there are few trials. The I^2 value is a more sensitive way of examining heterogeneity: 0% indicates no heterogeneity and 100% a high degree of heterogeneity.[4] In Figure 8.1, I^2 is 19.1%, which is low. On this occasion, the conclusion based on I^2 is consistent with the test for heterogeneity.

It is useful to investigate heterogeneity, because the overall effect may not be meaningful if the effect sizes clearly differ between trials. When there is significant heterogeneity that can be explained by a certain factor (e.g. trials conducted on younger people have a different effect size than those among older people), the effect size in each sub-group of the factor might be a more appropriate estimate of treatment effect than the overall estimate.

8.5 Considerations when reading a systematic review

There are several aspects of any review to consider when deciding whether it provides good evidence for or against a new intervention.

Differences in disease definition, the interventions and outcome measures

Trials are conducted in different ways using a variety of methods, and therefore the definition of the disorder, the outcome measures, and the delivery of the intervention may all vary between trials. In the trials in Figure 8.1, the control group consisted largely of smokers who had placebo gum, but sometimes the control group were those who were offered standard smoking cessation therapy, usually by counselling. It is not always possible to easily combine trials in a systematic review, particularly if the designs are very different. However, different trials that produce similar results may provide some evidence that a new intervention is effective, because the difference in methodology should increase variability, making it more difficult to find a treatment effect. It is also useful to determine whether the chosen endpoints are appropriate for addressing the objective of the review, when deciding whether a particular trial should be included.

Identifying studies

Systematic review reports should provide sufficient information on how studies were identified, by specifying the search criteria employed. This includes the range of years in which articles were published, whether foreign language articles were excluded, and which databases were used (e.g. Medline and Embase). More specifically, appropriate keywords should be used when searching the databases. In a review of a cancer treatment, it is insufficient to search using only the word 'cancer', because some abstracts use 'tumour' or 'carcinoma'. Different spellings should also be considered, for example 'randomised' and 'randomized', and some reports refer to patients who are 'randomly allocated' rather than 'randomised'. This can be partly overcome by using wildcards, i.e. the search term would be 'random*', where the asterisk allows for any letters after 'random'. If many studies are missed, the review may not be representative, and the results could be biased.

Publication bias

Trials with negative results (those contrary to what is expected, or those reporting no evidence of an effect) are sometimes less likely to be published than those that do show an effect, either because the research is not submitted for publication, or because journals reject them. In this situation, the pooled effect size from the meta-analysis will be biased towards the positive studies, and be larger than the true value. There are statistical methods that can detect significant publication bias. A simple method is a **funnel plot**, which plots the effect size against the weight (or 1/standard error, or standard error), and if the spread of the observations is clearly asymmetric, this is evidence of possible publication bias.[5]

Study quality

After the articles for a review have been identified, study quality may be assessed, and those judged to be inferior excluded from the meta-analysis. Exclusion could be based on an assessment of the study design, conduct or analysis, with consideration of potential bias or confounding. Even if the criteria for exclusion are clearly defined, this is a subjective exercise that could produce a biased selection of studies to be used in the analysis. If a particular trial is affected by bias or confounding, consideration should be given to whether the effect is likely to be so large that it clearly distorts the results. When assessing the effect of study quality it is perhaps best to include all trials, and then perform the analysis after excluding those considered 'poor quality'. Results can be compared to see how consistent they are.

Reporting systematic reviews

It is important that the way systematic reviews were conducted are reported clearly so that health professionals can judge the reliability of the results and conclusions. A report based on a systematic review should include the following items, though a more detailed set of guidelines can be found in Moher et al:[6]

- The main objective
- The search strategy, including the search terms and electronic databases used, as well as other sources of clinical trials
- How full articles were selected for inclusion in the meta-analysis; including specification of the target population, the disorder, the trial endpoints, and the interventions
- Specifying the total number of abstracts found during the electronic search, how many full articles were examined, how many were used in the meta-analysis, and how many were excluded, and the reasons for their exclusion
- A table summarising the main characteristics of each trial used in the meta-analysis, such as geographical location, time period when the trial was conducted, sample size, subject population (e.g. age range and gender distribution), the interventions and the effect size
- Method of statistical analysis (fixed or random effects model), the effect size used, and any investigation of heterogeneity if it exists, such as a formal statistical test or I^2 value
- Interpretation of the results, and their implication for clinical practice.

8.6 Why systematic reviews are important

An example of how meta-analysis could have affected medical practice sooner than it did is given in Figure 8.3. The left side of the figure shows the individual odds ratio of dying (similar interpretation to relative risk) for 33 randomised trials comparing intravenous streptokinase with a placebo or no therapy in patients who had been hospitalised for acute myocardial infarction.[7] Of the trials, 25 suggested a beneficial effect of streptokinase, but only six had a statistically significant result. The combined treatment effect showed that the risk of dying was reduced by about 25%, which was highly statistically significant. Of greater importance is the figure on the right-hand side. This is a **cumulative meta-analysis**. Each observation represents the pooled treatment effect of all the published trials up to that point in time. For example, the dot at 'European 2' is a meta-analysis of this trial and the three preceding ones. This figure shows that if a meta-analysis had been performed in the mid 1970s, a clear effect on mortality would have been observed. However, intravenous streptokinase was only recommended in the 1990s. The work on streptokinase took place before systematic reviews were common. Had such a review been conducted in the 1970s streptokinase could have been shown to be life saving almost 20 years earlier, long before its actual adoption into clinical practice.

Conventional and cumulative meta-analysis of 33 trials of intravenous streptokinase for
acute myocardia infarction. Odds ratios and 95% confidence intervals for effect of treatment on
mortality are shown on logarithmic scale

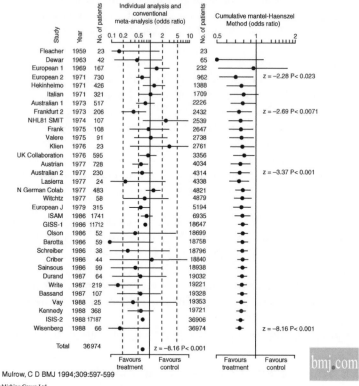

Figure 8.3 Meta-analysis of trials of streptokinase (reproduced from Mulrow 1994).[7] Reproduced
with kind permission from the BMJ Publishing Group.

8.7 Key points

• Systematic reviews are based on a formal approach to obtaining, analysing
and interpreting all the available studies on a particular topic
• A meta-analysis combines all relevant studies to give a single estimate of
the effect size, which has greater precision than any individual trial
• The conclusions from a review are usually stronger than those from any
single study.

References

1. Tang JL, Law M, Wald N. How effective is nicotine replacement therapy in helping people
   to stop smoking? *BMJ* 1994; **308**:21–26.
2. DerSimonian R, Laird N. Meta-analysis in clinical trials. *Controlled Clinical Trials* 1986;
   7:177–188.

3. RevMan Analyses (Computer program). Version 1.0 for Windows. In: Review Manager (RevMan) 4.2. Copenhagen: The Nordic Cochrane Centre, The Cochrane Collaboration, 2003. http://www.cc-ims.net/RevMan
4. Higgins JPT, Thompson SG, Deeks JJ, Altman DG. Measuring inconsistency in meta-analyses. *BMJ* 2003; **327**:557–560.
5. Sterne JAC, Egger M, Davey Smith G. Systematic reviews in health care: Investigating and dealing with publication and other biases in meta-analysis. *BMJ* 2001; **323**:101–105.
6. Moher D, Cook DJ, Eastwood S *et al.* for the QUORUM Group. Improving the quality of reports of meta-analyses of randomized controlled trials: the QUORUM statement. *The Lancet* 1999; **354**:1896–1900.
7. Mulrow CD. Systematic Reviews: Rationale for systematic reviews. *BMJ* 1994; **309**:597–599.

Further reading on systematic reviews and meta-analysis

Published articles

Davey Smith G, Egger M, Phillips AN. Meta-analysis: beyond the grand mean? *BMJ* 1997; **315**:1610–1614.

Egger M, Davey Smith G. Meta-analysis: potentials and promise. *BMJ* 1997; **315**:1371–1374.

Egger M, Davey Smith G. Meta-analysis: bias in location and selection of studies. *BMJ* 1998; **316**:61–66.

Egger M, Davey Smith G, Phillips AN. Meta-analysis: principles and procedures. *BMJ* 1997; **315**:1533–1537.

Egger M, Davey Smith G, Schneider M, Minder CE. Bias in meta-analysis detected by a simple graphical test. *BMJ* 1997; **315**: 629–634.

Egger M, Schneider M, Davey Smith G. Meta-analysis: spurious precision? Meta-analysis of observational studies. *BMJ* 1998; **316**:140–144.

Glasziou P, Irwig L, Bain C, Colditz G. *Systematic Reviews in Health Care: A Practical Guide.* Cambridge University Press, 2001.

Books

Egger M, Davey Smith G, Altman D. (Eds). *Systematic Reviews in Health Care: Meta-analysis in Context*, 2nd edn. BMJ Books, 2001.

Khan KS, Kunz R, Kleijnen J, Antes G. *Systematic Reviews to Support Evidence-based Medicine: How to Review and Apply Findings of Healthcare Research.* Royal Society of Medicine Press Ltd, 2003.

CHAPTER 9

Health-related quality of life and health economic evaluation

Previous chapters focus on clinical endpoints associated with efficacy and safety. However, it is also possible to examine new interventions from the subject's perspective, and in relation to financial costs. This chapter presents these two useful features of clinical trials. A trial team might have one or more members with this type of expertise.

9.1 Health-related quality of life

Common trial endpoints have a clear clinical impact, such as the occurrence or recurrence of disease, death, side-effects and changes in biological, biochemical or physiological characteristics. While these are usually taken to be the primary trial endpoints, it is sometimes useful to examine the effect of a new intervention from the subject's own experience, referred to as **health-related quality of life (QoL)**. Indeed, some equivalence or non-inferiority trials aim to show that a new intervention may have a similar clinical effect on the disorder of interest, but QoL is improved. QoL could, therefore, be one of the main endpoints. Most QoL measures are obtained through questionnaires, completed by the trial subject, guardian or relative, or during an interview with a health professional.

There is no fixed definition of QoL, but it aims to provide a quantitative measure of some or all of following:
- Pain
- Physical functioning
- Mental and emotional functioning
- Social functioning
- Feeling of well-being.

A new intervention with more side-effects may increase a patient's life by three months, but this could be balanced against the lower quality of life associated with the side-effects.

Elements of QoL and toxicity (or safety) often overlap. For example, pain level is specifically recorded in many treatment trials in advanced disease, but it may also be sought in QoL questionnaires. Perhaps the main difference

A concise guide to clinical trials, First edition. By A. Hackshaw. Published 2009 by Blackwell Publishing, ISBN: 978-1-4051-6774-1.

between some QoL measures and toxicity is that QoL is based on self-reported responses by the subject, and this is done in relation to several other factors, while toxicity is usually diagnosed by or with a clinician. There may not necessarily be a high correlation between QoL and toxicity.

Measuring QoL

There are many QoL questionnaires, sometimes referred to as **QoL instruments** or **measures**. Some have been developed for use in the general population, while others are intended for people who have a specific disorder. There is no perfect measure, and it is possible that when an instrument is used it will miss some important aspect of the subject's experience.

QoL responses are based on an individual's perceived experiences. These perceptions will vary between people, and also over time within the same person. It not unusual for QoL scores using different instruments to not be well correlated when completed by the same subject.

In choosing a QoL instrument for a trial, it is necessary to determine whether it will measure what subjects would consider important in that trial, and whether it is sensitive enough to detect meaningful changes in QoL. If many subjects report a very low (or very high) QoL score at baseline, there is not much scope to get a lower (or higher) score after treatment – called a floor (or ceiling) effect.

A **validated** QoL instrument is one that has been assessed and judged to measure what it is supposed to measure. The following questions are typical in making this judgement:

- Are the self-reported scores highly correlated with relevant objective or clinical outcomes? For example, if patients report high pain scores do they also request, or use, more pain relief medication?
- Do the scores from a QoL instrument correlate with scores from another, perhaps well-established instrument, both of which aim to measure similar aspects of QoL?

Reliability can be assessed by judging whether a QoL instrument will produce similar scores when repeated in similar groups of people.

Box 9.1 shows some QoL instruments used in research studies. Subjects usually rate their experiences or feelings on a scale. The Short Form 12 or 36 (12 or 36 questions) are commonly used measures.[1] For example, one of the SF-12 questions is: 'During the past four weeks, how much did pain interfere with your normal work (including both work outside the home and housework)?'

Subjects select only one of the following five responses: 'All of the time', 'Most of the time', 'Some of the time', 'A little of the time', or 'None of the time'.

These responses can be used to produce QoL scores in several **domains**. For example, the SF-12 has domains that include physical functioning, body pain, mental health and general health.

Other instruments, such as the EuroQol-5D (EQ-5D)[2] and the Health Utilities Index Mark 2 or 3 (HUI2 or HUI3),[3,4] aim to identify a subject's **health**

Box 9.1 Examples of QoL instruments used in clinical trials

General population

- Short Form 12 or 36 (SF-12 or SF-36)
- Nottingham Health Profile
- General Health Questionnaire (GHQ-30)

Disease-specific

- EORTC* QLQ C-30 (all cancer patients) and cancer-specific modules
- Parkinson's Disease Questionnaire
- St George's Respiratory Questionnaire (SGRQ)
- Dermatology Life Quality Index (DLQI)
- Stroke and Aphasia Quality of Life Scale (SAQOL-39)

Psychological

- Hamilton Anxiety Scale (HAS)
- Hospital and Anxiety Depression Scale (HADS)
- Psychological General Well-Being Index (PGWBI)
- Mental Health Index.

*EORTC: European Organisation for Research and Treatment of Cancer

---

state. These measures were often used with other QoL measures, but they are now used on their own. They can be used to estimate 'quality adjusted life years' (see page 152). For example, the EQ-5D covers mobility, ability for the subject to care for themselves, ability to undertake usual activities, level of pain and discomfort and mental health (anxiety and depression). One of the EQ-5D questions is:

'Please indicate which statement best describes your own health state today':

Mobility	I have no problems in walking about
	I have some problems in walking about
	I am confined to bed.

How many QoL instruments and how often?

Several different QoL instruments are used in some trials, often because results will be compared with those from previously published papers on the same topic. Because these reports were based on different measures, researchers believe they need to include most of them. When several questionnaires are planned, it is uncertain whether patients will complete them all or do so accurately, especially if one or more of the questionnaires contain many items. There is often overlap in the types of questions asked.

The timing of the measures depends on the natural course of the disorder of interest, and when detectable changes in QoL are expected to occur. For example, in a treatment trial of advanced lung cancer where most patients die within 1–2 years, it might be useful to collect QoL scores from patients every three months. In a disease prevention trial among healthy subjects, one QoL measurement annually might be sufficient. Asking subjects to complete questionnaires frequently has the advantage of allowing a better examination of how QoL changes over time, but this may not be feasible.

In determining the number and frequency of QoL measures, trial subjects should not be faced with too many pages to fill in, and not too often. This is especially important if the trial subject is ill. Either situation could be off-putting and so result in missing data. It may be better to have complete or near-complete data from one or two well-timed questionnaires than lots of missing data from several questionnaires, or a situation where the subject chooses not to submit any responses at all.

Analysing QoL scores

QoL instruments contain several questions. A total score for each subject can be obtained by simply summing the individual scores. Alternatively, the score from one question, or a group of questions, is summed separately, to provide a value for one of several domains. The score for each subject is often transformed onto a scale that ranges from 0 to 1 (or 0 to 100). Detailed instructions on how to deal with raw scores, and transform them, are usually provided with the instrument.

Table 9.1 shows three questions from the SF-12. Each response is assigned a value 1 to 5. The values are ordered categorical data: a score of 4 means the subject feels better than someone with a score of 2, but it cannot be said that they feel twice as good.

QoL scores can come under the category 'taking measurements on people' (see page 21). When comparing the average scores between two intervention arms, allowance must be made for the baseline score. When presenting QoL data, the mean baseline scores (or median if the distribution is skewed) and standard deviation indicate the scores before treatment starts.

If the mean baseline values are similar, the simplest analysis is to take the difference between the QoL score at one timepoint, say six months, and at baseline in Treatment Arm A (D_A), and to do the same in Treatment Arm B (D_B). A relevant and important time point should be chosen, i.e. long enough for the effect of the trial treatment to appear. The effect size is D_A minus D_B, and corresponding confidence intervals and p-values can be calculated (see page 98).

Table 9.2 illustrates this using QoL endpoints from a placebo-controlled trial evaluating thalidomide in addition to standard chemotherapy, in treating lung cancer patients. Thalidomide had no effect on global health status and the functional scales, but patients on thalidomide suffered less insomnia and more constipation (both are expected effects of this drug).

An alternative analysis is to compare the proportion of subjects with a high score (e.g. 4 or 5) between the trial arms, and use methods associated with 'counting people' (see page 91). However, information on variability is lost by turning a continuous measurement into categorical one.

Table 9.1 QoL responses for a trial subject using three questions from the SF-12.

	All of the time 1	Most of the time 2	Some of the time 3	A little of the time 4	None of the time 5
Q3. During the past four weeks, how much of the time have you had any of the following problems with your work or other regular daily activities as a result of your physical health?					
a) Accomplished less than you would like	X				
b) Were limited in the kind of work or other activities			X		
Q5. During the past four weeks, how much did pain interfere with your normal work (including both work outside the home and housework)?					X

Q3 (a) and (b) are combined to give a score for the domain 'Role physical'

Raw score = sum of the observed scores = $1 + 3 = 4$

Transformed score = [(raw score − lowest possible score)/ score range] × 100 = $(4 − 2)/8 × 100 = 25\%$

Q5 on its own is used to give a score for 'Bodily pain'

Raw score = observed score = 5

Transformed score = [(raw score − lowest possible score)/ score range] × 100 = $(5 − 1)/4 × 100 = 100\%$

Table 9.2 Summary data on selected quality of life domains based on the EORTC QLQ-30[5] in a trial comparing thalidomide with placebo in treating lung cancer patients; results at about six months after randomisation.

Domain	Mean score at baseline[a] (standard deviation)		Mean difference (six months - baseline)		Effect size	
	Placebo N = 318	Thalidomide N = 331	Placebo $Diff_P$	Thalidomide $Diff_T$	Mean difference (99% CI)[b] $Diff_T - Diff_P$	p-value
Global health status	50 (26)	49 (24)	+8.1	+9.9	+1.8 (−5.9, +9.6)	0.54
Functional scales						
Physical functioning	62 (27)	61 (25)	+4.2	+5.2	+1.0 (−6.8, +8.9)	0.74
Role functioning	49 (36)	48 (35)	+10.1	+10.0	−0.1 (−10.2, +10.0)	0.98
Social functioning	60 (34)	61 (32)	+8.0	+9.5	+1.5 (−8.1, +11.0)	0.70
Symptom scales						
Insomnia	50 (35)	48 (36)	−19.8	−31.7	−11.9 (−22.4, −1.3)	0.004
Constipation	27 (35)	29 (33)	−7.7	+3.0	+10.7 (+1.0, +20.6)	0.005

Data from personal communication (Dr Siow Ming-Lee, University College London Hospital)

[a]The scores range from 0 to 100 for all endpoints. For the global health and functional scales 0 indicates poor health and 100 good health. For the symptoms scales, 0 indicates no symptoms and 100 high level of symptoms.

[b]For the global health and functional scales a positive difference indicates that thalidomide was better and a negative difference indicates that placebo was better. For the symptoms scales, a negative difference indicates that thalidomide was better and a positive difference indicates that placebo was better.

Repeated assessment of the same QoL measure

When the instrument has been completed on several occasions, for example, there is a value for nausea at baseline, 6, 12 and 18 months after randomisation, an analysis could be performed at each time point. However, if this is done too many times, the presentation of results may appear unwieldy, and it might be difficult see what is happening. This analysis ignores the fact that a subject has contributed several QoL data points during the trial, and that these are likely to be correlated. Also, as more time points are examined separately, this increases the chance of finding a spurious effect.

If the QoL values for one measure from each subject were plotted against time, the result would be a 'curve' consisting of connecting straight lines (Figure 9.1). One way of analysing this is to calculate the **area under the curve**, so that there is only one data value for each subject. This allows statistical methods for 'taking measurements on people' to be used (Chapter 7). There are also advanced statistical methods that allow a single analysis of all the individual data points from all subjects (**repeated measures analysis** or **mixed modelling**). Analysing the whole data set in this way avoids having to look at multiple time points.

Having several comparisons

There are often several comparisons, each corresponding to a specific domain (Table 9.2 has six comparisons). The more comparisons examined from the same trial, the more likely it is that a spurious effect is found (see page 115). Adjusting p-values for having multiple comparisons might be considered,

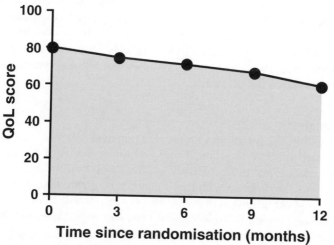

Figure 9.1 Example of a quality of life score profile for a single trial subject. Measures were taken at baseline, 3, 6, 9 and 12 months. The QoL scores at each of these time points are 80, 75, 72, 68 and 61%. The area under the curve is 70% (the example is in Table 9.4).

such as the Bonferroni correction (see page 115). However, some QoL scores are likely to be correlated, so this approach would make the p-value larger than it should be. Alternatively, the unadjusted p-values and 99% confidence intervals might be presented, as in Table 9.2, with caution given to p-values that are just under the conventional cut-off of 0.05, because this does not provide good evidence for an effect. Strongest effects are found when $p < 0.001$.

Some QoL instruments can be reduced to one or two domains. For example, the 12 questions on the SF-12 reduces to eight domains, which could be reduced further to two ('physical' and 'mental'), thus avoiding having several comparisons. However, there could be treatment effects on specific domains, which are masked when they are aggregated.

Missing data

Consideration should be given to how to handle missing data, because there could be reasons for this that bias the results, such as more subjects in one trial arm who were too ill to complete the questionnaires. If the proportion of subjects with missing data and the reasons for missingness are similar between the trial arms, the results are unlikely to be biased. When estimating effect sizes at a single time point (say 12 months) a subject who has only provided QoL data at six months presents a dilemma. They are unlikely to retrospectively complete the 12-month form reliably (unlike many clinical endpoints which could be obtained from hospital files retrospectively). This subject could be excluded from the analysis or the six-month value could be used as the 12-month value (referred to as 'last value carried forward'). Neither approach is perfect, but both are simple. There are also statistical methods called **imputation** which involve estimating what the subject's value might be, perhaps based on other data from the subject or data from other trial subjects. Methods such as mixed modelling use whatever data is available, without the need for imputation, though this assumes that missing data is randomly distributed between the trial arms.

Type of analysis

Where possible, an intention-to-treat (ITT) analysis should be performed, as is standard practice for clinical trial endpoints. For equivalence or non-inferiority trials a per protocol analysis could also be conducted (see page 116). However, the problem with trial subjects who do not take their allocated treatment (non-compliers) is that while it may be possible to obtain information on clinical endpoints from hospital files, and so include them in an ITT analysis, it is unlikely that QoL data will be available. If the subject has chosen to stop treatment, they may also decide not to complete any further trial forms. Consideration should then be given to whether there is a high proportion of non-compliers and if there is a potential for bias in the observed results, if this differs between the trial arms.

Interpreting QoL scores

QoL measures are subjective, and as such could be affected by trials in which
the allocated intervention is known. When interpreting QoL data, consideration should be given to the possible effect of the lack of blinding.

Treatment efficacy using effect sizes such as risk difference, relative risk
and number needed to treat, can often be described in a way that many people understand. For example, the reduced chance of developing a disorder,
or increase in survival time. However, one of the challenges with using QoL
results is how to translate them into practice. For many subjects or health professionals it may be difficult to interpret a specified difference in scores. For
example, how would a difference of −11.9 points for insomnia be interpreted
by a patient (Table 9.2)? Also, how much worse is a mean difference in constipation of −20 compared to −10 points? Describing the effect as small, medium
or large could be one way of summarising the average beneficial and negative
effects, without trying to interpret the actual effect size.

9.2 Health economic evaluation

In most societies, financial resources for health care are limited. With advances
in medical treatments, and an ageing population in many developed countries, governments need to monitor how much to spend on public health
and hospital services. Health economic evaluation is therefore an increas-
ingly important consideration when investigating a new intervention, especially with the rising costs of many new drugs, for example, in cancer. Cost-
effectiveness analysis is often used as a broad description for an economic
evaluation, but the term has a more specific meaning.

Several countries have processes for evaluating the cost-effectiveness of
new interventions. How they do this depends on the health care system in
place. Examples of institutions that perform these types of analyses are the US
Food and Drug Administration, the National Institute for Health and Clinical
Excellence (NICE, UK), Haute Autorité de Santé (HAS, France) and the Institute for Quality and Efficiency in Health Care (IQWiG, Germany). On the basis
of an evaluation of efficacy and health economic costs, these institutions may
choose which interventions to recommend for routine use. It is possible that
some treatments, although effective, are not recommended because they are
judged to be too expensive in relation to the clinical benefit.

What is economic evaluation?

There are three features of an economic evaluation in a trial:
- There is a comparison between two or more interventions, even if the
  comparison group received no intervention
- The treatment effect on a clinical endpoint(s)
- The costs, particularly financial costs, associated with the interventions.

The purpose is to consider both treatment efficacy and costs, and to determine whether or not a new intervention is more cost-effective than another

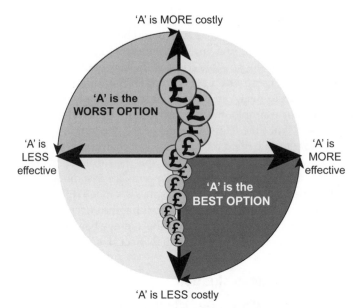

Figure 9.2 Comparing the effectiveness and financial costs of a new intervention (A) with an alternative (e.g. standard) treatment. The horizontal axis could be the effect size (e.g. risk difference, or difference in QALYs), and the vertical axis could be the difference in financial costs between the interventions.

intervention (Figure 9.2). It is not the case that the cheapest treatment is always recommended. The treatment of choice is likely to be both cheaper and more clinically effective. However, side-effects and QoL may also be considered. A treatment that is both less effective and more expensive would not be recommended. If two interventions have a similar effect, then the choice might be based on costs. Difficulty arises when the treatment is more effective, but more expensive (NE quadrant of Figure 9.2), in which case it is necessary to determine whether the extra costs are worth the improvement in efficacy. Similarly, if an intervention is less costly but less effective (SW quadrant), is the loss of efficacy justified by the cost savings? In both these situations, there may need to be a trade-off.

Types of economic evaluation

Costs in an economic evaluation are measured in monetary values, and generally fall into the following categories:

- Cost to the service provider (hospital or health service) of administering the interventions (e.g. treatment cost, cost of assessments or hospital stay)
- Cost to the subject (e.g. travel to hospital)
- Societal costs (e.g. number of work days lost).

The first of these is perhaps the easiest to obtain, because it is associated with clearly defined items, such as the cost of a drug, X-ray, blood test or treatment for a drug-related toxicity. The costs of such services are often obtained from published list prices, nationally available costs or the internal estimates from organisations, such as a hospital. The other two categories can cover a wide range of activities, including valuing lost days of work due to illness, or inconvenience to the subject if they have to travel to a hospital to receive a new treatment. Allocating a monetary value to some of these activities may not be easy. Many health economic evaluations concentrate on the cost to the service provider. It is also usual practice to standardise financial costs in the future to what they might be in present day values, allowing for inflation. The effect of discounting is small when the costs and health benefits occur at the same time, but large when costs could be incurred over many years. Annual discount rates are typically 3–6%. For example, a cost of £5,000 per year over 25 years corresponds to a total of £125,000 if unadjusted, but it becomes £68,000 if discounted using a fixed annual rate of 6%.

Four methods of health economic analyses are presented below, though the first two are the most commonly used. Many trials now collect subject-level cost data, i.e. there is a cost estimate for treatments and/or assessments for each trial subject.

Cost effectiveness analysis

When clinical efficacy is expected to differ between two interventions, unit costs can be considered in relation to the clinical outcome. One intervention is recommended over another if it is cheaper and more effective. But when the better treatment is more expensive the **incremental cost-effectiveness ratio** could be examined. This is illustrated in Table 9.3, based on a hypothetical randomised trial comparing two interventions (A and B). The number of deaths at one year is the main endpoint. The extra cost associated with saving five more lives is £20,000 using Treatment A, or £4,000 per extra life saved. Whether this is worthwhile is a judgement made by the service provider, who may also consider whether the same money could be invested elsewhere but with a greater benefit.

Other examples of incremental cost-effectiveness ratios are cost per year of life gained, or cost of detecting/diagnosing one extra affected individual, in trials of screening and diagnostic tests. This analysis allows comparisons

Table 9.3 Example of a simple cost-effectiveness analysis.

	Intervention A	Intervention B	Absolute difference (A minus B)
Number of subjects treated	500	500	
Number of deaths at one year	15	20	–5
Total cost of treating the group of subjects	£30,000	£10,000	£20,000

$$\text{Incremental cost-effectiveness ratio} = \frac{\text{difference in costs}}{\text{difference in efficacy}} = \frac{20,000}{5} = £4,000$$

between different medical areas if it is possible to express these in the same unit of measurement (e.g. cost per life year saved). It is also possible to use 95% confidence intervals for the cost-effectiveness ratios, using methods such as bootstrapping.

Cost utility analysis

This type of analysis incorporates quality of life measures. The financial costs of two interventions are compared with the outcomes measured in **utility-based** units. The most commonly used measure is the Quality Adjusted Life Year (QALY), which allows both the number of years and quality of life gained associated with a new intervention to be examined. Questionnaires such as the EQ-5D, SF-6D, HUI2 or HUI3 allow QALYs to be calculated. This is illustrated in Table 9.4. When there are several values from different time points, the area under the curve is used to calculate the total QALY for each subject.

A QALY for one year is in the range 0 (death) to 1 (perfect or full health). A subject can occasionally consider some states to be worse than death, so the value could be less than 0. A QALY of 0.7 means that the subject's quality of life is worth 0.7 of a year of full health. In Table 9.4, the subject's QALY for the first year is given, but values for subsequent years can be summed. For example, if the total over three years were 2.5, the subject has experienced 2.5 QALYs out of a possible total of three. If a new treatment extends a subject's life for one year, but at half full health it is associated with an increase of 0.5 QALYs (1 × 0.5). If life is extended by three years at half full health there is an increase of 1.5 QALYs (3 × 0.5).

Suppose two interventions, A and B, are compared in a trial, and each subject's health state is obtained over several time points (as in Table 9.4). Every subject has an 'area under the curve' value, and the mean area under the curve

Table 9.4 Calculating a QALY for one trial subject who has provided four EQ-5D responses in one year (i.e. every three months) in addition to the baseline value.

Month of EQ-5D	EQ-5D score	Time period (months)	Calculation[a]	QALY
0	0.80			
3	0.75	0–3	(0.80 + 0.75)/2 × 0.25	0.19
6	0.72	3–6	(0.75 + 0.72)/2 × 0.25	0.18
9	0.68	6–9	(0.72 + 0.68)/2 × 0.25	0.17
12	0.61	9–12	(0.68 + 0.61)/2 × 0.25	0.16
Total				0.70[b]

[a]The calculation involves taking the average of two consecutive QoL scores then multiplying by the time interval in years (3 months is 0.25 years)
[b]This is the area under the curve for this subject (the calculation is simple when the time interval between responses is the same throughout)

is obtained in each trial group: Mean_Area$_A$ and Mean_Area$_B$. There are also the financial costs of administering the interventions to the subjects in groups A and B: Cost$_A$ and Cost$_B$ (e.g. the mean cost in each group). An incremental cost-effectiveness ratio can then be calculated, similar to that mentioned above:

$$\text{Ratio} = \frac{\text{Cost}_A - \text{Cost}_B}{\text{Mean\_Area}_A - \text{Mean\_Area}_B} \quad \text{e.g.} \quad \frac{£25,000 - £10,000}{3.2 - 1.5} = \frac{£15,000}{1.7}$$

The result, £8,823, is the cost per one QALY gained (i.e. the marginal cost), and it indicates how much it costs to gain an extra year of healthy life using the new intervention. This is a common measure used in economic evaluation, and it allows health service providers to compare different interventions for the same disorder, and also interventions in unrelated areas of medicine.

Service providers often produce guidelines on what might be considered to be a cost-effective intervention, based on the cost per QALY gained. For example, the National Institute for Clinical Excellence in the UK, does not look favourably on interventions with a cost per QALY gained that far exceeds a specified amount (£20,000 to £30,000 in 2008).[6]

There are also analytical methods that allow for variability in the effect size and in the financial costs (for example, bootstrapping), producing a range of costs per QALY gained, similar in principle to confidence intervals. This method of economic analysis is preferred by many organisations that conduct health technology assessments because it incorporates quality of life, based on a common outcome measure, and can produce a range of estimates that indicates the uncertainty around the decision to adopt a new technology.

Cost minimisation analysis

When two interventions are expected to have a similar clinical efficacy, the decision on which to choose may rest on financial costs; i.e. what is the cheapest treatment. There should be evidence from equivalence trials. The effect size, such as relative risk, hazard ratio or difference between two means, should fall within a relatively narrow window around the no effect value. This method of analysis is not often used because it does not easily allow for variability in treatment effects or costs. Also, it is better to consider efficacy and costs together, as in the approaches given above.

Cost benefit analysis

In a cost benefit analysis, all outcomes are valued in monetary terms, including treatment efficacy. Subjects are asked to estimate how much they would be willing to pay for a certain increase in health (e.g. one extra year of life) associated with a new intervention. This could then be directly compared with the costs that arise from the intervention (e.g. costs to the health provider). However, there are several difficulties with this approach, including subjects having to understand the full implications of having the new intervention or not, and that willingness to pay may vary greatly between subjects. It is therefore not a commonly used method.

9.3 Summary

- It sometimes useful to examine the effect of a new intervention from the subjects' perspective
- Health-related quality of life (QoL) attempts to quantify various attributes such as mental and physical well-being
- When conducting a trial, consideration should be given to the number of different QoL instruments used, and how often subjects are expected to complete them
- As more interventions are developed, there is a need to have health economic evaluations, particularly where there are limited financial resources
- Several methods of analysis are available, but cost-utility analysis is commonly performed. It produces a financial cost per quality of life year gained, and allows different interventions to be compared.

References

1. Ware JE, Kosinski M, Turner-Bowker DM, Gandek B. *How to score Version 2 of the SF-12 Health Survey.* Quality Metric Inc., Lincoln, RI 2002. http://www.qualitymetric.com/
2. The EuroQol Group. EuroQol – a new facility for the measurement of health-related quality of life. *Health Policy* 1990; **16**:199–208. http://www.euroqol.org/
3. Torrance GW, Feeny DH, Furlong W *et al.* Multi-attribute preference functions for a comprehensive health status classification system. Health Utilities Index Mark 2. *Med Care* 1996; **34**:702–722.
4. Feeny DH, Furlong W, Torrance GW *et al.* Multi-attribute preference functions for a comprehensive health status classification system. Health Utilities Index Mark 3. *Med Care* 2002; **40**:113–128.
5. Aaronson NK, Ahmedzai S, Bergman B *et al.* The European Organisation for Research and Treatment of Cancer QLQ-C30: A quality-of-life instrument for use in international clinical trials in oncology. *J Nat Cancer Inst* 1993; **85**:365–376. http://www.eortc.be/home/qol/
6. National Institute for Health and Clinical Excellence. http://www.nice.org.uk/

Further reading

Heath-related quality of life

Addington-Hall J, Kalra L. Who should measure quality of life? *BMJ* 2001; **322**:1417–1420.
Carr AJ, Gibson B, Robinson PG. Is quality of life determined by expectations or experience? *BMJ* 2001; **322**:1240–1243.
Carr AJ, Higginson IJ. Are quality of life measures patient centred? *BMJ* 2001; **322**:1357–1360.
Farsides B, Dunlop RJ. Is there such a thing as a life not worth living? *BMJ* 2001; **322**:1481–1483.
Fayers P, Hays R. *Assessing quality of life in clinical trials.* 2nd edn. Oxford University Press, 2005.
Fayers PM, Machin D. *Quality of life: assessment, analysis and interpretation.* John Wiley & Sons, Ltd, 2000.

Higginson IJ, Carr AJ. Using quality of life measures in the clinical setting. *BMJ* 2001; **322**:1297–1300.

Spiegelhalter DJ, Gore SM, Fitzpatrick R *et al.* Quality of life measures in health care. III: resource allocation. *BMJ* 1992; **305**:1205–1209.

Streiner DL, Norman GR. *Health measurement scales*. 3rd edn. Oxford University Press, 2003.

Health economics

Byford S, Raftery J. Perspectives in economic evaluation. *BMJ* 1998; **316**:1529–1530.

Byford S, Torgerson DJ, Raftery J. Cost of illness studies. *BMJ* 2000; **320**:1335.

Glick HA, Doshi JA, Sonnad SS, Polsky D. *Economic evaluation in clinical trials*. Oxford University Press, 2007.

Palmer S, Byford S, Raftery J. Types of economic evaluation. *BMJ* 1999; **318**:1349.

Palmer S, Torgerson DJ. Definitions of efficiency. *BMJ* 1999; **318**:1136.

Raftery J. Economic evaluation: an introduction. *BMJ* 1998; **316**:1013–1014.

Raftery J. Costing in economic evaluation. *BMJ* 2000; **320**:1597.

Robinson R. Economic evaluation and health care: What does it mean? *BMJ* 1993; **307**:670–673.

Robinson R. Economic evaluation and health care: Costs and cost-minimisation analysis. *BMJ* 1993; **307**:726–728.

Robinson R. Economic evaluation and health care: Cost-effectiveness analysis. *BMJ* 1993; **307**:793–795.

Robinson R. Economic evaluation and health care: Cost-utility analysis. *BMJ* 1993; **307**: 859–862.

Robinson R. Economic evaluation and health care: Cost-benefit analysis. *BMJ* 1993; **307**: 924–926.

Robinson R. Economic evaluation and health care: The policy context. *BMJ* 1993; **307**:994–996.

Torgerson DJ, Byford S. Economic modelling before clinical trials. *BMJ* 2002; **325**:98.

Torgerson DJ, Campbell MK. Use of unequal randomisation to aid the economic efficiency of clinical trials. *BMJ* 2000; **321**:759.

Torgerson DJ, Campbell MK. Cost effectiveness calculations and sample size. *BMJ* 2000; **321**:1697.

Torgerson D, Raftery J. Measuring outcomes in economic evaluations. *BMJ* 1999; **318**:1413.

Torgerson DJ, Raftery J. Discounting. *BMJ* 1999; **319**:914–915.

CHAPTER 10

Setting up, conducting and reporting trials

Setting up and conducting clinical trials is more difficult than it was several years ago, largely because of increased regulations and required governance responsibilities. This chapter summarises the clinical trial process (Box 10.1). Some sections only relate to trials evaluating a drug or medical device. Although details vary between countries, there are some fundamental similarities. Current requirements and timelines for regulatory and ethical approval should be checked [See page 185 for glossary of common terms].

10.1 Pre-trial

Establishing a working group and the trial team

A small multidisciplinary **working group** of key people (say three to five) should initially develop the project. They agree the trial objectives and endpoints, and share responsibility for writing the trial protocol and, perhaps, the grant application. The group should include relevant health professionals, a statistician and other speciality members, for example, trial co-ordinator, pathologist or health economist.

After securing funding, the group can expand to form the **trial team**, (also called **trial management group**, or **trial steering group/committee**) to manage the trial over its entire duration. It could additionally include expertise in data management, regulations and safety monitoring, IT (database and randomisation systems) and some investigators from the larger centres.

Estimate the financial costs of the trial

Clinical (especially multi-centre) trials can be difficult and expensive to set up and conduct. Staff funding and resources necessary for planning, trial initiation and conduct, follow up and statistical analyses should not be underestimated.

The number and type of staff required will depend on the complexity of the trial and sample size, and could include a trial co-ordinator, data manager, statistician, pathologist, laboratory technician, research nurse, health

A concise guide to clinical trials, First edition. By A. Hackshaw. Published 2009 by Blackwell Publishing, ISBN: 978-1-4051-6774-1.

Box 10.1 Key elements to the trial process

Pre-trial

Establish working group to develop idea
↓
Estimate the financial costs
Secure grant funding (when required)
↓

Trial set-up

Develop trial protocol, patient information sheet, consent form
↓
Obtain EudraCT number (EU only)*
Record trial on an international clinical trials register
↓
Obtain authorisation from regulatory authority
Obtain ethical approval
Implement procedures for drug handling
↓
Develop the case report forms
Develop the necessary agreements and contracts
Obtain approval from each site
Set up trial in centres (e.g. site assessment & initiation)
Activate sites
↓

During trial

Conduct trial; monitor progress in sites
Independent Data Monitoring Committee review
↓
Send annual safety report to regulatory authority*
Send Annual Progress & Safety report to Ethics Committee
↓

End of trial

Lock database
Close trial (inform regulatory authority*)
Sponsor & recruiting sites should store all relevant documentation
↓
Published first efficacy and safety results
↓
Long-term follow up (efficacy and/or safety)#

---

*Where required. This is usually only for trials investigating an investigational medicinal product
not always done

---

economist and someone with expertise in quality of life. The salary costs for staff will depend on how much time they will spend on the trial and where the work will be undertaken (central trials unit, and patient recruitment at centres). For example, large trials often require at least one full-time dedicated staff, but small trials, where there are few subjects recruited per month, should only require part of a person's time to manage the trial daily.

Other costs could include:
- Those to be met by recruiting centres: for example, extra clinical assessments, extra blood or tissue samples, pathological reviews or laboratory analyses
- Office and travel expenses; printing protocols and case report forms (page 171), and travel and other costs for the trial group meetings, centre initiation and monitoring visits (see pages 174 and 179)
- Applications to the regulatory authority, where necessary, and sometimes the independent ethics committee (see pages 167 and 169)
- A fee for each patient recruited, sometimes required by centres.

Secure funding

Therapies evaluated by the manufacturer, for example, pharmaceutical companies, usually have internal funding. Non-commercial organizations, such as universities, hospitals or public sector departments, must usually seek external funding. Grants to conduct clinical trials may come from governmental bodies, charities and private benefactors, but funds are limited and competitive. Although the format of the application forms will vary, many aspects are often covered by the trial protocol (page 161).

Funding bodies usually seek value-for-money, and may not look favourably on a small, very expensive trial. Dividing the total grant requested by the expected number of subjects gives a crude cost per subject. If this looks high, it is worthwhile justifying clearly why the resources are essential. Many funders specify what costs they will not cover, for example, a new drug from a pharmaceutical company. It is worthwhile listing centres that have already agreed, in principle, to participate.

A grant application is more likely to succeed if the trial has the potential to change practice, or sometimes to provide further valuable information on a disorder, perhaps leading to larger studies. It should be produced by a working group that has discussed key issues thoroughly, so that these are not picked up for the first time by the funding committee or their external reviewers.

Do the interventions need regulatory approval?

Many regulations focus on trials of an investigational medicinal product (IMP, in the EU), or investigational new drug (IND, in the US or Japan). Classifying a trial drug as an IMP, or not, determines the paperwork required to obtain the approvals and which systems must be in place during the trial. Generally, a substance, or combination of substances, is an IMP if the trial aims to determine whether it affects disease treatment, detection or diagnosis, or prevent disease or early death (see pages 2 and 190). In some countries, it may also include substances used to restore, correct or modify physiological functions (e.g. in the EU). An IMP could be a new drug that is not licensed for human use, or one that already has a marketing authorisation. Some countries have

---

Box 10.2 Sponsor and investigator

• Sponsor: An individual, company, institution or organisation which takes responsibility for the initiation, management and financing of a clinical trial. The sponsor must ensure that the trial is conducted in accordance with any relevant regulations and guidelines.

• Chief investigator (CI): A single named person responsible for the trial design and conduct, though the sponsor has ultimate responsibility. The CI is often the person who conceived the idea for the trial or may be a key opinion leader in the disease area. He/she is named as the lead investigator on applications for regulatory and ethical approval. The CI often works in the same institution that acts as the sponsor.

• Investigator: A person who is responsible for conducting the trial at a site (centre). Where a group of people are involved in trial conduct at the site, one person should be identified as the principal investigator (PI).

---

additional legislation relating to certain medical devices and exposures such as radiotherapy. The local regulatory authority can advise on this.

10.2 Trial set up

Many research departments have the primary purpose to design, set up and analyse clinical trials, and this work is central to pharmaceutical companies. These organisations have permanent staff in place, including clinicians, statisticians, trial co-ordinators and IT personnel. Where there is limited direct access to such resources, it is advisable to seek advice.

Identify the lead trial researcher, sponsor and recruiting investigators

A **Sponsor** is the institution with ultimate responsibility for the trial design and conduct (Box 10.2). An individual is rarely the sponsor because of the legal, insurance and indemnity implications. The **chief investigator** is the key researcher for the trial, and often first developed the idea. A **principal investigator** is an individual responsible for the trial at a single recruiting centre.[#]

It is usually easy for multi-national commercial companies to sponsor international trials if they operate with legal status in the relevant countries. However, a university, for example, acting as a sponsor does not normally have a legal status in another country. Certain responsibilities of trial conduct and safety monitoring must therefore be delegated to named individuals or institutions in each foreign country, and this would need to be specified in an agreement (see page 172).

[#] chief investigator and principal investigator are not standard terms, but their roles are.

Many pharmaceutical companies employ an independent commercial **contract research organisation (CRO)**, to conduct the trial on their behalf. The pharmaceutical company remains the named sponsor, but many of the responsibilities are delegated to the CRO.

Potential recruiting centres, often called **sites**, should be identified, with a realistic estimate of the number of expected subjects per site (investigators tend to over-estimate this). This helps ensure that the target sample size is feasible in a reasonable timeframe.

Trial protocol

The protocol provides justification for the trial, details of the design, and a set of instructions for sites and the co-ordinating centre, describing how subjects are to be recruited, treated (with the trial interventions and other treatments, where necessary) and followed up, and the systems in place for safety monitoring. It ensures the trial is conducted to a similar standard across all sites and it ultimately reduces variability, making it easier to find a treatment effect if it exists. The protocol is signed off by the sponsor and chief investigator.

While some trial protocols can be up to 20 pages, those for IMP trials are often longer, because they require more details on trial conduct, administration of treatments and safety monitoring. The protocol should contain a clear plan of what will happen to subjects, from the time they consent to participate to the time they leave the study. For non-drug trials (e.g. surgical interventions, or changes in behaviour or lifestyle), it is important to describe the delivery of the intervention clearly in the protocol, to ensure consistency and standardisation across the trial. Table 10.1 shows suggested key sections in a protocol, Figure 10.1 shows a simple flow diagram giving an overview of the trial, and Table 10.2 is an example of how to summarise the timing of assessments.

The objectives (aims) of the trial should not be confused with the endpoints. The outcome measure is quantifiable and used to address the objective (Box 10.3). There should be one, at most two or three **primary objectives**, each associated with an endpoint. Other objectives and endpoints should be referred to as **secondary**. The primary endpoint is the one that would change practice.

The wording of the objectives should be consistent with the phase of trial. Phase I and single-arm phase II studies are often easy to describe. However, the wording for a randomised phase II trial may make it look like a phase III trial. Phase II studies only provide preliminary evidence on the effectiveness of a new intervention, so the objective could use words such as 'to examine' or 'to investigate', to avoid suggesting that the trial results will conclusively show whether the new treatment works or not. For phase III trials, stronger words such as 'to evaluate', 'to show' or 'to determine' (Box 10.3), are perhaps more appropriate.

Patient information sheet and consent form

All subjects, or their legal representative (see page 191), must give informed consent before participating in a clinical trial. Sufficient information about the

Table 10.1 Suggested sections in a trial protocol.

Section Heading	Description
Chief investigator and Sponsor	• Name and address of one individual who is the overall lead, and the representative of the institution acting as the sponsor
	• Both need to sign and date each version
The trial management group	• The names, affiliations and roles of members of the trial team
Background to the trial	A fairly concise summary of:
	• The scale of the disease burden (e.g. prevalence or incidence)
	• The effect of current interventions
	• Reference to trials or systematic reviews that are relevant to the proposed trial
Justification for the trial	• A summary of why a trial is needed now, and how it may be expected to change practice, or be used to justify further studies
	• The current evidence and biological plausibility for the new intervention
Trial design	• Type of trial – phase I, II or III; randomised or single-arm; single- or double-blind
Objectives	• There should be one or two primary ones (used to determine whether health practice should change), and possibly several secondary ones (that would provide additional information)
Outcome measures	• There should be primary or secondary endpoints, each corresponding to the specified objectives
Sample size	• There should be enough information for the sample size to be reproduced independently, with reference to the expected treatment effects from published or unpublished work, or an effect that is the least clinically important
Target population	• A list of inclusion and exclusion criteria (see page 11)

Interventions	• A clear description of what the trial interventions are and how they will be administered, including the dose and frequency (if applicable) and duration of treatment • Other treatments to be given at the same time should be specified • If free drugs or medical devices are supplied, from say a pharmaceutical company, this should be stated with a summary of how they will be supplied, documented and where appropriate, destroyed
Recruitment and Follow up	• The length of the recruitment and follow-up periods should be specified • When added together they should represent the total length of the trial • Many trials will specify an 'active' phase, which ends when the last patient has completed the last protocol visit, after which the follow-up phase begins
Assessments of subjects	• A detailed description of how subjects will be assessed – how frequently, what will happen at each visit (such as clinical examinations, tests and any other evaluation), and how long subjects will be in the trial
Case report forms (see page 170)	• A list of what they are, when they should be administered (Table 10.2) and who should complete them (the subject or researcher)
Safety monitoring	• A list of any known expected adverse reactions associated with the trial treatments • Describe the procedures for identifying, monitoring and reporting all adverse events
Consent and trial approvals	• Summarise the procedures for obtaining informed consent, and ethical and regulatory approval
Statistical analyses	• A description of the main statistical methods to be used to analyse the main and secondary endpoints • Specification of the analyses that would be based on intention-to-treat or per-protocol • Specification of subgroup analyses • If there are any planned interim analyses, specify how they will be used
Insurance and indemnity	• Mention what cover is in place if a subject is harmed through participating in the trial
Ownership	• A statement about ownership of the trial data

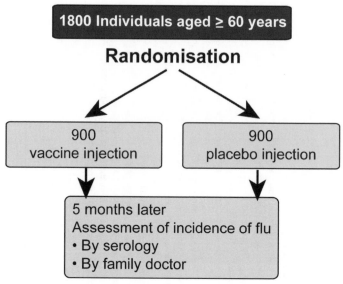

Figure 10.1 Example of a flow diagram of a trial of a flu vaccine.

trial should be provided to allow them to examine the possible benefits and risks of taking part. Information may be provided verbally, or by video, DVD or audio tape, but it should always be given in writing: the **patient information sheet** (PIS). After reading this, subjects must sign and date a **consent form**, which is co-signed by an authorized staff member. Suggested sections are shown in Boxes 10.4 and 10.5. Signed consent forms should be kept in the site files, and a copy given to the patient.

The text in these documents should be clear and written in simple language. Additionally, there may be site- or country-specific requirements, such as insurance, or they may need to be translated into another language (see page 193). It is often useful to ask a few subjects or members of a patient

Table 10.2 Example of a table that summarises the timing of assessments.

	Baseline	Intervention period			Follow up	
		3 months	6	12	18	24
Assessments[a]						
Subject history	X					
Clinical examination	X	X	X	X	X	X
Blood sample	X			X		X
CT scan	X			X		
Other case report forms (CRFs)						
Quality of life	X		X	X		X

[a]there should be a CRF to record this information as it is collected; for example, six clinical examinations should yield six CRFs.

Box 10.3 Examples of descriptions of objectives and endpoints

Phase of trial	Objective	Outcome measure (endpoint)
I	To determine the maximum tolerated dose of a new therapy for advanced colorectal cancer	The number of patients who suffer a dose-limiting toxic event
II	To investigate Drug A in patients with Parkinson's disease	The proportion of patients who progress after one year
II	To examine the potential effect of Therapy B for lung cancer	The proportion of patients who have a partial or complete tumour response
III	To evaluate the effectiveness of a flu vaccine in the elderly	The proportion of people who develop flu
III	To determine the effectiveness of statin therapy in people without a history of heart disease	Mean serum cholesterol level
III	To show whether a Therapy D for asthma has a similar effect as standard treatment	The proportion of patients who suffer a severe asthma exacerbation.

representative group to comment on the text before it is finalised, particularly for complex trials or those with several arms. Both the PIS and consent form should be signed off by the sponsor and chief investigator. The independent ethics committee (see page 169) may recommend changes.

The subject should be neither encouraged nor discouraged to participate. When discussing the trial with an eligible subject, the health professional should try to maintain a position of equipoise, i.e. there is genuine uncertainty over the effect of the new intervention. Sometimes this is difficult to do. For example, in surgical trials, the patient expects the surgeon to recommend the best treatment. Here, it might be better for a non-surgeon to discuss the study.

In IMP and medical device trials, subjects could be given a card to carry showing their unique trial number, a brief description of the trial and 24-hour contact details of trial staff or site representatives. This is common in blind trials.

EudraCT number (EU IMP trials only)

The EudraCT (EU Drug Regulating Authorities Clinical Trials) database contains information about all IMP trials conducted in the EU. Before regulatory or ethical approval can be sought, a EudraCT number (a unique identifier) must be obtained via the European Medicines Agency (EMEA).[1]

Box 10.4 Recommended sections in a patient information sheet

- Background and justification for the trial
- A description of how subjects will be randomised, and the probability of being in each treatment arm
- A description of the trial interventions, especially identifying those that are experimental
- What the trial subject has to do as part of the trial and the expected duration of their participation
- Which tissue samples, if any, are being collected, and what will be done with them for the purpose of the trial and for future research
- What are the possible side-effects of the interventions (including the magnitude of the risks, and discomforts to the subject, as well as to any embryo, foetus or nursing infant of the subject)
- The possible benefits and disadvantages of taking part
- Alternative procedures or treatments available to the trial subject if they do not participate
- A statement about securing confidentiality of subject data and who will have access to the data
- A statement that participation is voluntary and refusal to participate will involve no penalty or loss of benefit; and that the subject may withdraw at any time
- Circumstances under which a subject's participation may be terminated by the investigator without regard to the subject's consent
- Who is funding the research
- Who to contact if there are any queries, including a 24-hour telephone number in an emergency
- A statement about liability and compensation if something goes wrong.

Register the trial

All trial reports, not just those with 'positive' results, should be published. To minimise the bias associated with researchers not submitting 'negative trials', or journals not publishing them, there are international systems of clinical trial registration. All new trials should be recorded on a recognised database before recruitment starts. This has been a legal requirement in the US since 2007, and sponsors of marketing applications must certify that they have complied.[2] Common trial registers are:

- International Standard Randomised Controlled Trial Number (ISRCTN) (http://www.controlled-trials.com/)
- www.ClinicalTrials.gov.

These databases contain information about the main objectives, design, outcome measures, duration and funding. They allow researchers to check on other trials in progress or that have been completed. Many medical journals require the registration number when considering an article for publication.

Box 10.5 Examples of text used in a consent form

• I confirm that I have read and understood the information sheet Version 1.0 dated 10 January 2008.
• I understand that my participation is voluntary and that I am free to withdraw at any time, without giving any reason and without my medical care or legal rights being affected.
• I understand that my medical notes may be looked at by responsible individuals or by regulatory authorities* where it is relevant to my taking part in research. I give permission for these individuals to have access to my records.
• I give permission for an extra blood sample to be taken at the start of the trial. I understand that giving this sample is voluntary and that I am free to withdraw my approval for its use at any time without giving a reason and without my medical care or legal rights being affected.
• I agree that the blood sample I have given, and the information gathered about me, can be stored at *Institution's name* for use in future studies.
• I agree for my family physician to be told of my participation in this study.
• I agree to participate in the trial.
• Signature of the trial subject or legal guardian.

*these could be listed, for example, trial monitors, trial co-ordinator, regulatory authority, etc.

Regulatory approval (for certain interventions)

In most countries, the clinical trial regulations specifically cover IMP or IND (i.e. drug) trials, and sometimes medical devices. Before recruitment can begin, regulatory authority approval must be obtained in each country in which the trial will be conducted. The sponsor and chief investigator (Box 10.2) must be named on the protocol, and applications to regulatory authorities and ethics committees. Each EU country has its own **Competent Authority** (CA), to issue regulatory approval. The equivalent body in the United States is the Food and Drug Administration (FDA), and in Japan it is the Pharmaceutical and Medical Devices Agency (see also pages 197 and 198).

For newly developed drugs, it is sometimes useful to meet with the regulators to reach agreement on the trial design. This is particularly so for phase III trials, which may be used later to make claims about effectiveness and contribute to a marketing authorization application. In the US, sponsors could arrange a formal meeting with the FDA.[3] In the EU, sponsors may seek scientific advice from the Committee for Proprietary Medicinal Products.

To gain regulatory approval, several documents must be submitted to the regulatory authority (Box 10.6): called the Clinical Trial Application (in the EU), or Investigational New Drug application (in the US).

The **Investigator's Brochure (IB)** provides detailed information about the trial drug, including:

Box 10.6 Examples of documents needed for submission for regulatory approval to conduct an IMP/IND trial

- The EudraCT number*
- Investigator's Brochure (IB); or Summary of Product Characteristics (SmPC)*
- Investigational Medicinal Product Dossier (IMPD)*
- Investigational New Drug (IND) application**
- Information about the investigators, recruiting sites and laboratories
- Details of drug manufacturing and distribution (e.g. Qualified Person documentation in the EU)
- Trial protocol and sample consent form
- Specification of measures to deal with vulnerable subjects, when required
- Completed application form
- Information about the independent ethics committee
- Fee.

*European Union Trials
**US Trials

- Its physical, chemical and pharmaceutical properties, with evidence from laboratory studies
- A description of the pharmacological, metabolic and toxicological results from animal experiments, and methodological details of these experiments
- A description of the metabolic, safety and efficacy evidence from studies of human subjects, such as phase I data, or marketing experience if the drug already has a licence
- An example of the drug label, from the manufacturer.

There should be one IB for each drug being evaluated, and it is not usually specific to a trial. The IB provides justification for the dose, method of delivery and other biological aspects of the IMP specified in the trial protocol, and describes the expected safety profile based on animal data and previous human experience. This allows the trial investigators to assess the possible risks and benefits of the drug. The IB is usually developed and updated by the drug manufacturer (annually, or when new significant information becomes available), with significant input from at least one clinician. The recommended sections in an IB are listed in ICH GCP guidelines.[4]

For IMPs already licensed for human use, and to be used within the terms of the marketing authorisation, the regulatory body may require a Summary of Product Characteristics (SmPC) instead of a detailed IB.

The **Investigational Medicinal Product Dossier (IMPD**; EU IMP trials) provides information about the quality, safety and use of all IMPs in the trial, including placebo or any other comparator. It allows the regulatory body to examine the possible safety and toxicity profile of the product(s). Some information will overlap with that in the IB, and so can simply be cross-referenced. Again, the SmPC may suffice for drugs already licensed for human use. Requirements for the IMPD differ between countries so the regulatory body should be consulted before submission.

In the EU, the regulatory authority aims to assess applications within 30 days, followed by five days to inform the applicant whether it has been approved or declined. Further information may be requested, which may extend the processing time up to 60 days. For some trials, for example, gene therapy, genetically modified organisms, or xenogenic cell therapy (live cells or tissue from animal sources to be given to humans), the approval process is longer. For trials to be conducted in more than one EU member state, an application has to be made to the competent authority in each state.

An **Investigational New Drug (IND) application** must be filed for trials involving US residents. The sponsor must submit information on manufacturing and quality control, pharmacology and toxicology data, and data from prior human studies (unless previously submitted) to the FDA. For an original IND application, a sponsor may not initiate the study until 30 days after receipt at the FDA. For subsequent studies under the same IND, the 30-day wait period is not required, although the sponsor proceeds with the study at risk. If concerns arise, particularly relating to safety, the FDA may place all or part of the trial on hold until the sponsor adequately addresses the concerns. Thereafter, the sponsor submits annual reports to the FDA on the status of the study, and to update the general investigational plan for the coming year.

Regulatory authorities require the current name of the principal investigator at each recruiting site (e.g. in both the US and the EU). All 'substantial amendments' to trial documentation and design, must be approved by the regulatory authority (see page 176).

Independent ethics committee approval

All proposed trials should be reviewed and approved by an Independent Ethics Committee (IEC). It examines the trial protocol, and any documentation intended for the trial subject, such as the patient information sheet, consent form and questionnaires. The committee considers:

- The scientific justification for the trial and its design
- Acceptability to subjects, including an assessment of potential harms and benefits
- The administrative aspects of the trial, including procedures for compensating trial subjects in case of negligence
- The suitability of the investigators.

The committee may request changes to the trial design, conduct or documentation. In the EU, the committee has a maximum of 60 days to approve or decline the application, and is permitted a single request for further information, which temporarily halts the 60-day period. There is sometimes a dialogue between the researchers and the committee if aspects of the trial need to be resolved.

Applications are stronger if the trial design has already had independent peer review, for example, through a grant application. Involvement of subjects or patient representatives in developing the patient information sheet and consent form could demonstrate that the wording is likely to be acceptable to potential trial subjects.

The process for obtaining ethical approval varies between countries and according to whether the trial is single or multi-centre. For single-centre studies a local ethics committee is appropriate. For multi-centre studies, 'national' approval might be possible. For example, applications in the UK are made to a single organisation via a website, and considered by one of several committees. Approved trials may be then conducted anywhere in the UK. In other countries, for example, the Netherlands, applications can be made to one of several organisations, but approval also allows the trial to be conducted throughout the country. In the United States, ethics is reviewed by an Institutional Review Board (see page 173), one at each recruiting site. Sometimes one IRB covers several sites.

Procedures for handling trial drugs

The sponsor has ultimate responsibility for how IMPs (or INDs) or other trial-specific treatments, including placebo and any other comparator drugs, are manufactured, transported, stored and processed during the trial. Several procedures need to be established (Box 10.7).

Requirements for handling IMPs differ between countries. In the US, the sponsor often deals with drug quality assurance, handling and distribution, or one of more of these functions may be delegated. In the EU, IMP manufacturers or importers must hold a **manufacturing authorisation**, granted through the regulatory authority. Only the authorised holder can be involved in production, import, assembly, blinding, packaging, labelling, quality control, batch release and shipping. A **Product Specification File** contains written instructions, or refers to other documents, used to perform these activities. At least one named **Qualified Person (QP)** should be responsible for the product specification file. They must sign a release certificate (**QP release**) for each batch and for the final product sent to sites or trial subjects. For IMPs imported into the EU, the QP must sign a QP release certificate, indicating that each batch meets the appropriate standards for Good Manufacturing Practice. A system may be needed to recall batches if there is a problem, particularly if drugs do not have a marketing license.

A manufacturing authorisation, QP and QP release are always needed for unlicensed drugs in the EU. For drugs that are already marketed for human use, these are required only if an organisation does something with the drug, or its packaging or labelling, as part of the trial. For example, in a double-blind trial with placebo, the drug name must be removed.

Case report forms (CRFs)

Data are always collected from trial subjects. This could come from clinical records, additional assessments and tests performed within the trial, or

---

Box 10.7 Procedures for quality assurance of IMPs (INDs) in clinical trials

The Sponsor should have documentation to ensure that:
- The drugs are manufactured in accordance with guidelines on Good Manufacturing Practice
- The drugs are stored according to the manufacturer's specification
- The drugs are packaged and shipped in such a way to prevent contamination and deterioration
- Individual packages are correctly labelled (including contact details of the sponsor or other trial team member, expiry date, an identifier, batch number and instructions to the trial subject on storage and administration, 'keep out of reach of children' for drugs to be taken at home and 'for clinical trial use only')
- The correct pack code is given to drugs in blind trials, and that the code for a particular pack can be unbroken in an emergency in some trials
- Drugs are delivered to sites or trial subjects in a timely fashion, and there is a clear system for ordering further supplies
- Each recruiting site keeps records on drug shipment (including dates and batch numbers) and receipt, and return and destruction of unused drugs
- Records are kept on biochemical analyses of sample batches
- Enough drugs will be available for the whole trial and target number of subjects
- Drugs batches can be recalled when necessary.

---

questionnaires completed by the subject. These data are used to evaluate treatment compliance, efficacy and safety. Trial-specific **case report forms** (CRFs) are an efficient way of collecting data because not all subject data will be useful for the trial. Examples of CRFs could be:
- *Baseline CRF:* Includes dates of birth and randomisation, the allocated intervention (or treatment code if the allocations are concealed), physical characteristics (e.g. weight and height), blood measurements, possibly an assessment of pre-treatment disease and confirmation that the eligibility criteria have been met.
- *Treatment CRFs:* Include details of trial interventions and other treatments received by subjects, how these were administered, which allocated trial interventions were not received and why.
- *Efficacy CRFs:* These collect variables that allow estimation of the treatment effect (and effect sizes), for example, date of disease occurrence or recurrence, or death; presence of absence of a disorder, characteristic or habit.
- *Safety CRFs:* These record variables associated with adverse events, including those that are expected. Enough space must be left for unexpected events to be recorded (this could be a separate CRF).

CRFs should be simple and relatively quick to complete, which will also reduce the time taken to enter the data onto an electronic database. This is particularly important for trials with long follow up, because recruiting sites usually have limited resources and the number of trials they are involved in is likely to increase over time. The CRFs should be developed by the trial team, so that all key variables directly associated with the efficacy endpoints, safety and treatment compliance are recorded. Phase I and II studies are exploratory and based on relatively few subjects, so many variables may be needed to obtain a clearer view of the potential safety and effectiveness of a new therapy, because this will decide whether it is investigated further. However, too many variables, particularly for large phase III trials, may result in complex or multiple forms. Many variables may not be used at all in the statistical analyses, and site staff may fail to ensure that key variables are completed. The CRF format may help to determine how the data will be analysed, and the structure of the electronic database.

Traditionally, CRFs are printed on paper, and completed by hand. These data are then entered, again by hand, onto a trial **database** (see page 177). However, some large organisations (e.g. pharmaceutical companies) use an **Electronic Data Capture (EDC)** system, where site staff record subject data electronically, directly onto CRFs on the computer screen. The data is then automatically stored in the central trial database. This minimises paperwork and possibly time spent processing subject data, though the electronic CRFs still need to be developed.

Agreements
The following agreements should be considered, though the names may differ between countries. National guidelines and the sponsor will specify which are necessary, and what details they need to contain. There are legal implications associated with fraud (falsifying trial subjects, or subject's data), negligence, lack of informed consent, insider trading, and withholding trial results (see also page 192).

Clinical trial (site) agreement
This is an agreement between the sponsor (often the co-ordinating centre) and each recruiting site, listing the roles and responsibilities of the sponsor, local investigator and sites. It is mandatory for EU IMP trials. It aims to ensure that the site must have the necessary regulatory and ethics approval in place before starting recruiting, and that it conducts the trial according to Good Clinical Practice, in particular handling the drug or medical device appropriately, ensuring subject safety and timely reporting of adverse events, and that all trial data is sent to the co-ordinating centre. It also specifies the sponsor's responsibilities, for example, data management and analyses of the data, and ensuring that the site is always informed of any relevant trial documentation and revisions. The agreement should also outline the responsibilities of the site pharmacy for handling and disposal of trial drugs. Specially adapted

agreements are usually required between the sponsor and international sites, and this can take several months to finalise because of issues over insurance, indemnity and which country's law takes precedence. It must clearly specify which tasks have been delegated to overseas sites. If part of the protocol is incorrect, a site may claim compensation from the sponsor if, for example, a subject has suffered harm as a consequence. Similarly, the sponsor may claim compensation from the site if, for example, subjects or data have been falsified. The agreement should state the amount of money to which each claim is limited.

Drug supply agreement
When a manufacturer has agreed to supply a free drug (and sometimes placebo), this needs to be documented, so that there is an obligation to continue supply for the target number of subjects. It is signed between the sponsor and manufacturer and certifies that they are operating to Good Manufacturing Practice (see page 195), and outlines the roles and responsibilities of the parties. Where a third organisation is involved in packaging or distribution, a tripartite agreement, or separate technical agreement (or quality agreement), may be acceptable.

Other service agreements
Technical or service level agreements may be needed between the sponsor and any other organisation providing services for the trial (e.g. pathology reviews and biochemical analyses). While they may not be legally binding, they ensure that all parties understand the detail and standards of the work to be undertaken.

Material transfer agreement
If biological samples (e.g. blood or tissue) are to be sent from a recruiting site to a central laboratory or depository (such as a tissue bank) for trial-specific or future research, an agreement may be required between the site and destination organisation, to ensure that, for example, samples are handled safely and stored appropriately. The ownership of the samples and rights to intellectual property arising from the research should be made clear. The sponsor may also wish to have a service agreement with the central depository to clarify the roles and responsibility of each party in relation to the biological samples.

Institutional approval

Sponsor
The institution acting as the sponsor will have its own internal review of the trial design, conduct, protocol, and assessment of subject safety and well-being. This is because it has ultimate responsibility for the trial and may have legal responsibility to financially compensate any subjects harmed by the trial. The sponsor must ensure that there is sufficient indemnity cover for this. Most

trials now need to have a named sponsor, whatever the intervention being tested.

Recruiting sites

All institutions from which subjects are to be recruited will review the protocol, documentation for subjects and, where appropriate, the Investigator's Brochure. This is because the institution will be partly responsible for conducting the trial to Good Clinical Practice, including ensuring that subjects have given informed consent, adverse events are being recorded and reported, drugs are received and distributed to subjects appropriately, and that trial data are sent to the co-ordinating centre. A clinical trial may incur local financial costs (e.g. additional X-rays or blood tests that are not part of routine care, or treatment costs) that would not be covered by a grant, so the site will need to agree to meet these.

Institutional approval may be conducted by a Research and Development committee in the UK. In the US or Japan an **Institutional Review Board (IRB)** is used, which may also evaluate ethics.

Site assessment and site initiation

Potential recruiting centres may be assessed by a member of the trial team (usually the trial co-ordinator) before or at the same time as institutional approval is sought: **site assessment**. This could involve visiting the site to examine the staff, systems and procedures in place for:
- Subject recruitment
- Storage and supply of trial drugs to subjects
- Administering the trial interventions and undertaking assessments
- Data collection and completion of case report forms
- Reporting of adverse events.

Multi-centre trials may list the minimum criteria for participating sites in the trial protocol. The purpose is to identify problems that may arise, and to judge whether the site is able to conduct the trial according to Good Clinical Practice (i.e. a form of **risk assessment)**. The assessment could be by a questionnaire to be completed by the site which confirms they are able to conduct the trial to a high standard. The main interest is in minimising possible risks to subjects in the trial, but also risks to the sponsor, who despite delegating certain responsibilities to the site, will bear ultimate responsibility for trial conduct over all recruiting sites.

Site initiation aims to familiarise local site staff with the proposed trial and the protocol, and to establish a link with the trial co-ordination centre. The trial co-ordinator may attend the site in person, or initiation may be performed by a teleconference, particularly for relatively simple trials. Site staff involved in the trial, and their delegated functions would be recorded.

Site assessment and initiation are common practices for multi-centre trials, and are useful for all IMP (IND) trials because of the regulatory requirements.

For small trials or non-drug studies, the extent to which these activities are carried out will depend on the resources available.

10.3 Trial conduct

The trial can proceed after obtaining the approvals and signed agreements. The Sponsor, Chief Investigator, and Co-ordinator should have access to a set of **essential documents**, which together form the **Trial Master File** (TMF, Box 10.8). A full list of documents in the TMF (held by the Sponsor) and Investigator File (held at each recruiting site) are identified in ICH GCP.[4] Having these kept in a single location, allows easy review and audit. During the trial, regular reports on progress and safety may be sent to oversight bodies (e.g. IRBs and regulatory agencies), who will specify what is required.

Box 10.8 Contents of a Trial Master File – suggested key Essential Documents

- Investigator's Brochure*
- Investigational Medicinal Product Dossier or SmPC*
- Approved trial protocol*
- Approved patient information sheet, consent form and any other documents for the subject*
- Case report forms (CRFs)*
- Financial aspects of the trial (e.g. letter from funder, insurance and indemnity cover)
- All signed agreements between sponsor, recruiting sites, drug supplier and other parties
- Approval letter and any correspondence with the sponsor from the regulatory agency
- Approval letters and any correspondence from all ethics committees/IRBs, including allowed advertising for subject recruitment and details of subject compensation, if applicable
- Approval letter from all recruiting centres
- Curricula vitae of the chief investigator and principal investigator from each site, and financial disclosure forms where applicable (to identify any potential conflicts of interest)
- Sample of labels for IMPs/INDs
- Product Specification File/QP release documentation
- Current laboratory certifications and laboratory normal ranges
- List of staff and their responsibilities.

*These need to be dated and have version numbers so that the most current ones can be identified easily.
A full list is given in Section 8 of ICH GCP.[4]

Recruiting sites should also keep documents such as the protocol, the patient information sheet, signed consent forms, a list of enrolled and screened patients with their unique trial numbers, and any other documents associated with trial set-up and conduct, for example, local approval documentation, site delegation logs and curriculum vita of site staff involved in the trial.[#] These should be contained in an Investigator Site File. For IMP trials, a site **Pharmacy File** could contain a list of the trial subjects and the drugs they received, staff delegation log, a summary of drug supply arrangements, records of drug receipt, dispensing and destruction, and any relevant local policies.

Many trials have dedicated staff to set up the study, collect and maintain all the documentation needed for the TMF, and monitor progress. This is in addition to helping with queries from sites and possibly subjects, entering and checking data and organising meetings of the trial team.

Changes to documents in the Trial Master File

The protocol, patient information sheet (PIS) and other documentation may change during the trial because of the following:

- Changes to the design, for example, the original eligibility criteria may be too strict and need to be relaxed
- New information from the published literature, the data monitoring committee, or interim reports may affect current or future trial subjects, so the PIS needs to be revised accordingly
- Additional data is to be collected so the CRFs must be revised
- The Investigator's Brochure should be updated annually, or when new significant information becomes available.

The regulatory authority should approve significant changes to the trial design or protocol, usually before being implemented. These changes, as well as those to documentation intended for subjects, should also be approved by the independent research ethics committee that gave the original approval, again before implementation. Once approved, updated information can be disseminated to sites. Significant changes could include anything that affects:

- The safety and well-being of the trial subjects
- The scientific value of the trial
- The conduct or management of the trial
- The quality and safety of any of the IMPs.

In EU trials, any significant change is referred to as a **substantial amendment**. All documents should have a version number and be dated.

Randomising subjects

An **eligibility checklist**, with each of the inclusion and exclusion criteria for a subject can be 'checked off' to make clear that the subject is eligible. This could

---

[#] Sites are legally obliged to keep some of these documents depending on the regulations in that country.

be a case report form, and copies are sent to the co-ordinating centre (see also page 85).

Statistical analysis plan (SAP)

At the start of the trial, the statistician could draft an outline of the statistical analyses to be performed at the end. This should include assessment of treatment compliance, efficacy and safety. It may be expanded after requests for interim analyses from the data monitoring committee during the trial (see page 179), but it should be finalized before the database is ready for the full analysis. A SAP avoids many unplanned analyses at the end of a trial, for example, many sub-group analyses. However, if there are important unexpected results, the SAP should not prevent an investigation of the data beyond the pre-specified analyses.

Database

All trial data should be entered onto an electronic database. For small non-randomised trials, a simple spreadsheet might suffice. For randomised, or large, trials it is better to use a proper database system, and there are several commercially available ones. This ensures that data entry is structured and makes researchers think more carefully about the data analysis. For IMP trials in the EU the database needs to be fully validated, and allow an **audit trail** of activity, where changes to the data are clearly recorded.

A problem with using a spreadsheet is that the same variable can be entered in different ways, and numbers and characters can be mixed together:

Date of randomisation	Body weight	Cancer type
03/01/2001	80 kg	Lung cancer
21/June/2005	187 pounds	Lung CA
15-Sep-2004	95 kg	Lung tumour

It is impossible to analyse this data. The dates all have different formats, weight is in a mixture of kg and pounds but it should only be in a single format with no text in the cells, and there are different spellings of the same disease. Statistical analysis packages would have difficulty reading this, and the data would require much manual editing before it could be analysed.

By using a dedicated database, computer screens can be made to look very similar to the paper CRFs, making data entry easier. Automated validation checks can minimise data entry error, or identify errors on the CRFs. For example, there could be an electronic check that the date of birth precedes the date of randomisation, and the trial treatment dates are after the randomisation date. Range checks could be used to identify extreme blood and physiological measurements. The database could also help identify overdue CRFs, or key variables that need to be chased up. It is important to ensure that information on the main efficacy endpoints and side-effects are as complete as possible, i.e. with minimal missing data, particularly for phase I and II trials.

Any database system must be securely stored, with access limited to relevant trial staff, and backed up regularly to minimise the amount of lost work if the system malfunctions. It should have a disaster recovery plan in place (e.g. in case of fire), and be sited on a robust IT network.

For double-blind trials, treatment allocation should only be visible in the database as a drug pack code so that trial co-ordinators and other trial staff with regular access cannot see which intervention has been allocated to each subject (see page 86). Only the trial statistician should be able to access this data for the purposes of the final analysis and interim reports to the data monitoring committee (see page 179).

Standard operating procedures (SOPs)

It is good practice for organisations involved in clinical trials to have a set of Standard Operating Procedures (SOPs). These are summary guidelines specific to the working practices of the organisation that show staff how to perform certain functions. They allow staff to conduct trials to the same standard, and new staff to quickly familiarise themselves with these practices. SOPs also show an external auditor or regulatory inspector that clear and robust systems are in place. Examples of SOPs are:
• Protocol writing
• Obtaining regulatory approval
• Obtaining ethical approval
• Initial site assessment (before recruitment)
• Setting up sites
• Randomisation procedure
• Database development and maintenance
• Recording and reporting adverse events
• Site visits during the trial
• Making and reporting protocol amendments
• Statistical considerations (sample size, statistical analysis plan)
• Closing the trial (chasing missing data, following up serious adverse events, ensuring that all the trial documentation is stored).

Meetings of investigators

In developing a new trial, the trial team should meet several times. This should continue during the trial, particularly in the early stages, to quickly identify and solve problems with recruitment, delivery of trial interventions, non-compliance or other key issues.

Investigator meetings are generally held for multi-centre trials with at least four or five sites. In phase II and III studies the principal investigator from each might be invited. The meetings are usually co-ordinated by the sponsor and, although they are not required by the regulations, they serve to educate and obtain consensus amongst the investigators on the design and conduct of the study, and train them on important elements of the study. Having meetings when all the sites are ready to start recruiting can also help motivate study personnel.

Regular newsletters to the investigators and staff at the recruiting sites detailing recruitment, and the amount of missing data that needs to be chased up, may be useful.

Monitoring of recruiting sites

The level of monitoring necessary for each study depends on its complexity and potential risks to the subjects or scientific validity of the trial. The sponsor will often assess this as part of the institutional review.

Monitoring could include checking that trial subjects really exist, that signed consent has been obtained, that data have been recorded correctly onto the case report forms (CRFs), and that adverse event reporting has been appropriate and timely. Pharmaceutical companies undertake a high level of on-site monitoring because they want their drug to be licensed, and regulatory authorities require clinical trials to be conducted according to ICH GCP guidelines (see Chapter 11). If the guidelines have been followed closely, an application for a license is less likely to be declined. **Source data verification (SDV)**, often conducted by pharmaceutical companies, involves checking some entries on the CRFs with what is contained in the patient hospital files. This can be done for all subjects (100% SDV) or a random proportion of them (e.g. 10% SDV). SDV can be an expensive activity, and there is uncertainty whether it noticeably changes the main trial results. Furthermore, data errors should be relatively uncommon but, more importantly, randomly distributed between the trial arms. However, the regulatory authority may indicate what it believes to be an appropriate level of SDV. Where the quality of data from a particular site is questionable, the trial team may decide that it requires SDV.

While pharmaceutical companies have the resources to monitor trials closely, non-commercial organisations may limit on-site monitoring activities to confirming that subjects are real and that there is signed consent. Central monitoring, using the electronic database, can identify errors on key variables. Formal statistical methods can also check data for, for example, digit preference, and compare a variable from one site with the average over all sites to detect outliers. The site would be contacted to correct or clarify identified anomalies. Central statistical monitoring is cheaper and easier to perform than full on-site monitoring and SDV.[5]

Independent data monitoring committee (IDMC)

This is a group (usually three to five people) of health professionals, a statistician and other relevant experts with no direct connection to the clinical trial. The IDMC provides an independent and unbiased review of the trial during the recruitment and treatment period, and advises the trial team. Key functions include:
- Safeguarding the interests of subjects
- Assessing safety and toxicity
- Identifying poor recruitment

- Monitoring the overall conduct of the trial, such as treatment compliance and missing data
- Examining data on efficacy.

The composition, roles and responsibilities of the IDMC, may be documented in a charter.[6] Before each meeting, the trial statistician, possibly with the trial co-ordinator, prepares a report for the IDMC, summarising several trial outcomes (see bullet points above). After reviewing the report, the IDMC will either support continuation of the trial, or make recommendations to close early. They may also request changes to the trial design, protocol, patient information sheet or consent form, if any of the trial data, or other evidence, indicates this is necessary. For double-blind trials, the report to the IDMC may conceal the interventions (for example, A and B to indicate aspirin and placebo), but the committee may request unblinded results if, for example, there is an imbalance in the number of adverse events.

The IDMC meetings can be in two parts. The open meeting, which the trial statistician, co-ordinator and other members of the trial team, such as the chief investigator, attend. They discuss issues associated with recruitment, collection of data and adverse event reporting (not according to trial arm). During the closed meeting only the trial statistician, who has produced the data on efficacy data by trial arm, attends. After the meeting, the IDMC will issue a report for the trial team.

If there is clear evidence that the trial should be suspended or closed early, the trial team and recruiting sites need to be informed quickly, particularly if there are concerns over safety.

Suspending or closing trials early

There may be several reasons why a trial must be temporarily stopped or closed early, for example, poor recruitment, unacceptable harm, a clear treatment effect was observed or futility (see page 122). The decision is usually made and agreed by the trial team and the IDMC. Systems need to be introduced to inform sites about recruitment and subjects already recruited, if the decision is likely to affect them directly, for example, a previously unknown increased risk of a disorder, or the subject needs to stop the trial treatment. The ethics committee, which originally approved the trial, should review and approve this information before it is sent to subjects. Where, for example, the trial has been stopped early because of poor recruitment it may not be necessary to contact subjects because those who are already in the trial could still be followed up as intended.

An important reason for suspending or closing trials early is patient safety. Sponsors in the EU (IMP trials) can implement **urgent safety measures** if there is an immediate significant risk to the health and safety of trial subjects. This can be done without first seeking approval from the regulatory agency or ethics committee, though these organisations need to be informed in writing, with clear justification, within three days. Urgent safety measures may be executed after discussion with the IDMC or a medical assessor at the regulatory authority. For all other reasons associated with early trial closure, either temporary or permanent, the sponsor must notify both the regulatory agency and ethics committee within 15 days, and give reasons.

10.4 End of trial

Trial closure may be implemented in two phases: closure of recruitment and closure of follow up. When the recruitment target has been reached, sites must be informed not to approach further potential subjects. This 'closure to recruitment' does not mean the end of the trial. The time point at which the trial should formally close is usually specified in the protocol. For example, this could be after the last recruited subject has been followed up for one year. The sponsor is usually required to notify both the regulatory authority and the ethics committee when this occurs (e.g. within 90 days in the EU for IMP trials). Trials may then enter a **long-term follow-up phase**, collecting key data on efficacy and safety for future evaluation. This too is specified in the protocol, but no notification is needed.

The status of the trial database should be examined and any missing key information on CRFs from sites should be sought. Once most of this data has been received and entered, the database is downloaded for statistical analysis, called **database lock**. This analysis forms the first full report.

The Trial Master File and the trial database should be kept by the sponsor for several years after the trial has closed (e.g. five years for IMP trials in the EU), and recruiting sites also need to keep relevant trial documentation and patient CRFs.

10.5 Monitoring adverse events

Identifying, recording and reporting adverse events are essential functions in trial conduct. The extent to which this is done depends on the intervention, for example, drugs, medical devices, surgery or behavioural changes. Monitoring drug safety is often called **pharmacovigilance**.

An **adverse event** is any untoward or unintended medical occurrence or response, whether it is causally related to the trial treatments or not. When it is judged that the event is likely to be caused by the intervention it can be called an **adverse reaction**, or **adverse drug reaction** in IMP trials. An adverse event could be the occurrence of a disease or condition that directly affects the patient's health, safety or well-being, including ability to function. It could also be an abnormal and significant biochemical or physiological measurement. Adverse events are not usually the same as the disease of interest, for example, if evaluating a new drug for advanced lung cancer, death from lung cancer is not classified as an adverse event, because it is an expected natural process for this disorder. Death from stroke would be considered an adverse event. However, if there are many more lung cancer deaths in the new treatment arm, stopping the trial early should be considered.

Adverse events and reactions can be **expected** or **unexpected**. They are expected when, for example, they are pre-specified in the marketing authorisation of a drug that is already licensed for human use, or the Investigator's Brochure or Investigator's Medicinal Product Dossier, if not licensed. Expected events should be listed in the trial protocol.

Adverse events or reactions, whether expected or unexpected, can be further classified as **serious adverse events (SAE)** or **serious adverse reactions (SAR)**, if any of the following occur:

- Death
- Is life-threatening
- Requires hospitalisation, or prolongs hospital duration if already in hospital
- Results in persistent or significant disability or incapacity
- Results in a congenital abnormality or birth defect
- Leads to any other condition, judged significant by the clinician.

They should normally be reported to the sponsor (or the co-ordinating centre) within 24 hours of discovery. An assessment must be made of whether the event is *suspected* to be causally related to the trial treatment and if it is *unexpected*: a **suspected unexpected serious adverse reaction (SUSAR)**. A SUSAR is the most important type of event, and requires special processing. If a trial is blind then assessment of causality and expectedness could be performed as though the patient were on the active treatment.

For IMP (IND) trials, a sponsor must report a fatal or life-threatening SUSAR to the regulatory authority within seven days of being notified.[7] If the SUSAR is not fatal or life-threatening, the regulatory authority must be informed within 15 days. The system and timelines are similar in many countries, including the EU, the US and Japan. The ethics committee or IRB which originally approved the trial must also be informed, usually within the same timeframe. The sponsor must also submit an Annual Safety Report to the regulatory authority, which includes:

- An analysis or summary of subject safety in the trial
- A list of all suspected SARs (expected or unexpected) to date
- A summary table of the suspected SARs.

When an SAE occurs in a trial with blinding, the treatment allocation may need to be revealed. This is almost always the case with a SUSAR, though usually only the person who reports the event, often the trial co-ordinator, would know the treatment allocation, and not the clinician or trial staff in the site from which the subject came. The treating clinician may need to be unblinded if it will affect how the subject is treated.

A system may need to be in place for **emergency unblinding**. The request for unblinding should come from the subject's clinician, or from a hospital to which the subject has been urgently admitted. During office hours, the trial co-ordinator or other named trial staff would be contacted. At other times, a member of staff from the co-ordinating centre who is 'on call', or the hospital pharmacy, should have access to the treatment allocation codes. For international trials, it may be possible to unblind directly through the electronic trial database though this system would need to be set up carefully and securely to avoid unnecessary unblinding. The decision to unblind must be clearly justified and a trial clinician should be involved if possible.

Whatever system for unblinding is implemented, there is likely to be a cost and resource issue. For trials investigating a drug that is unlicensed for human use, it is usually clear why emergency unblinding is needed. The justification may be less clear for common drugs, for example, a trial in adults to investigate whether aspirin could prevent cancer, though a case could be made if a child has accidentally taken the drug. If an SAE occurred, the clinician would and should treat the symptoms, without necessarily waiting to find out the trial treatment. Unblinding could take place the following working day. The need for a system for unblinding outside of office hours will depend on the disease and treatments being investigated, an assessment by the sponsor, and ultimately the requirements of the regulatory authority. There may also be a need to have access to **24-hour medical cover**, where a clinician treating the subject can seek information about the trial and the treatments being evaluated.

When the request to unblind is not associated with safety, relatively few reasons are likely to be justified. The decision should then be made for each individual, and agreed by the chief investigator or other members of the trial team. A system for this type of review could be provided in the protocol. It is important that the scientific validity of the trial is not adversely affected by unnecessary unblinding.

10.6 Reporting clinical trials in the literature

Results of all trials should be reported, usually in a health professional journal. There are detailed reporting guidelines (CONSORT).[8–11] The following main sections should be covered, though some parts may not be relevant to phase I or single-arm phase II trials:

Trial design and conduct
• Summarise the design (e.g. phase I, II or III; whether randomised or not; single arm or multi-arm; single- or double-blind; crossover; factorial)
• Specify who was blind to treatment allocation (the clinician giving the treatment, those assessing the subject, or the subject)
• Specify the method of randomisation (simple, stratified or minimisation) and state any stratification factors used, and block size
• Specify the inclusion and exclusion criteria
• Provide details of the sample-size calculation
• Specify how long patients were followed up for before the main outcome measure was assessed
• Specify how many randomised patients were later found to be ineligible

• Specify the proportion of patients in each arm who were not available for follow up (i.e. for whom the main trial endpoint is unavailable, i.e. withdrawals)
• Mention the methods of statistical analysis.

A diagram (called the CONSORT flow chart) could be provided, showing the number of eligible and ineligible patients randomised, the number allocated to each intervention, the number who complied with treatment, the number followed up and the number used in the statistical analysis. These are all reported for each trial group.

Interventions
• Describe the trial interventions being compared, including dose, frequency, duration and method of delivery
• Mention any other treatments given to patients at the same time.

Results
• State where the trial was conducted, the number of recruiting centres and calendar years of study
• Provide a summary table of baseline characteristics for each trial arm (without p-values)
• Provide summary measures of efficacy (effect size, 95% confidence intervals and p-values); including survival curves if using time-to-event endpoints
• Provide a summary of any side-effects observed, and whether they differed between the trial arms.
• For Phase I studies provide details of the pharmacological effects

Treatment compliance
• Define compliance and specify the proportion of patients in each arm who did not comply with the allocated trial treatments
• If there is a clear difference between these proportions, provide reasons (e.g. side-effects).

Discussion
• Mention any limitations of the study design or analysis
• Are the results consistent with other studies? If the results are unexpected, it is useful to provide possible explanations (e.g. the subjects had less or more severe disease than originally anticipated)
• What does the trial contribute to practice?

Most journals restrict the number of words, tables and figures, so researchers have to address the sections listed above concisely. This can be partly achieved by presenting results in a table rather than in the text. However, many journals are now available electronically, via the Internet, allowing supplementary text, tables and figures that do not appear in the printed version still to be publicly available. Covering all the sections listed above makes it more likely that journal editors and external reviewers will give a favourable view, because they are able to assess the paper properly.

Conflict of interests

Many publishers require a declaration of financial support received for a trial, any relevant patents and any connection with the manufacturers of products or devices used. Conflict of interests, sometimes referred to as competing interests, arises when the professional judgement concerning the validity and interpretation of research could be influenced by financial gain, or professional advantage or rivalry. Financial interests offer an obvious incentive to present a treatment in a more positive light.

Authors should state who funded the trial because this may have influenced their interpretation of the data, perhaps subconsciously. Sometimes, the interpretation is more in favour of one intervention than the results seem to support, or the conclusions indicate that the results are more generalizable than they really are. Authors should also declare any personal financial interests associated with the paper, including fees they may have received from manufacturers of the trial interventions, allowing the reader to judge whether this may have affected the trial conduct and interpretation of the results.

10.7 Summary

- Researchers should have clearly defined systems in place for trial set-up and conduct
- Many trials (usually drugs) require approval from the regulatory authority in each country from which subjects will be recruited
- All trials should obtain independent ethical approval and institutional approval
- Sponsors of trials should ensure that all the necessary documents, contracts and agreements are in place before recruitment begins
- There should be clear systems for identifying and reporting adverse events, particularly serious events
- Trial reports should contain all the necessary details on design and analysis, with a statement about competing interests.

Glossary of common terms

CA	Competent Authority
CI	Chief investigator
CRF	Case report form
CTSA	Clinical trials site agreement
EU	European Union
FDA	Food and Drug Administration (in the United States)
GCP	Good Clinical Practice
IB	Investigators Brochure

ICH	International Conference on Harmonisation
IDMC	Independent data monitoring committee
IMP	Investigational Medicinal Product
IMPD	Investigational Medicinal Product Dossier
IND	Investigational New Drug
IRB	Institutional Review Board
MTA	Material transfer agreement
QP	Qualified Person
PI	Principal investigator
PIS	Patient information sheet
SAE	Serious adverse event
SAR	Serious adverse reaction
SDV	Source data verification
SmPC	Summary of Product Characteristics
SOP	Standard Operating Procedure
SUSAR	Suspected unexpected serious adverse reaction
TMF	Trial master file

References

1. http://eudract.emea.europa.eu/
2. http://www.fda.gov/oc/initiatives/advance/fdaaa.html#actions
3. http://www.fda.gov/cder/guidance/2125fnl.htm
4. http://www.ich.org/LOB/media/MEDIA482.pdf
5. Baigent C, Harrell FE, Buyse M, Emberson JR, Altman DG. Ensuring trial validity by data quality assurance and diversification of monitoring methods. *Clin Trials* 2008; **5**:49–55.
6. Damocles Study Group. A proposed charter for clinical trial data monitoring committees: helping them to do their job well. *The Lancet* 2005; **365**:711–722.
7. http://www.mhra.gov.uk/Howweregulate/Medicines/Licensingofmedicines/Clinical trials/Safetyreporting-SUSARsandASRs/index.htm
8. Moher D, Schulz KF, Altman DG. The CONSORT Statement: Revised recommendations for improving the quality of reports of parallel-group randomized trials. *Ann Intern Med* 2001; **134**:657–662.
9. Campbell MK, Elbourne DR, Altman DG. CONSORT statement: extension to cluster randomised trials. *BMJ* 2004; **328**(7441):702–708.
10. Piaggio G, Elbourne DR, Altman DG, Pocock SJ, Evans SJW. Reporting of noninferiority and equivalence randomized trials: An extension of the CONSORT statement. *JAMA* 2006; **295**:1152–1160.
11. Ioannidis JP, Evans SJ, Gotzsche PC *et al.* Better reporting of harms in randomized trials: an extension of the CONSORT statement. *Ann Intern Med* 2004; **141**(10):781–788.

CHAPTER 11

Regulations and guidelines

There are various regulations and guidelines that are associated with setting up and conducting a clinical trial. However, the number and depth of detail often appear overwhelming to researchers, especially those new to research. This chapter provides an overview of the key issues covered by these regulations and guidelines, some of which were mentioned in Chapter 10. Most laws only cover drugs and some medical devices. For further details or current requirements, researchers should check their national guidelines, and consult their institution or regulatory authority.

11.1 The need for regulations

Clinical trials are experiments on humans. Subjects who participate are given an intervention that they would not normally receive, and they often undergo additional clinical assessments and tests, including having to complete questionnaires. They agree to participate for the planned length of the trial, which could be several years. It is therefore essential that their safety, well-being and rights are protected. This is the main purpose of the regulations and guidelines. They also ensure that the clinical trial data are valid and robust, and can be used to reliably demonstrate that the benefits of the intervention outweigh the possible risks. This is a critical component in providing assurance that the drug or medical device will be approved by regulatory authorities for use in the wider disease population.

Regardless of what regulations or guidelines are in place, researchers have an ethical and moral duty to be responsible for the subjects, and should be accountable to a higher body if subjects are harmed as a result of participating in the trial.

The first internationally recognised guideline was the Nuremberg Code[1] developed in 1948 after several German clinicians and administrators were prosecuted for conducting experiments on concentration camp prisoners without their consent (the Nuremberg Trials). Many prisoners suffered great pain, died or were permanently disabled. The Nuremberg Code formed the basis of the Declaration of Helsinki, developed by the World Medical Association (1964).[2] After several revisions it now consists of 32 paragraphs that

A concise guide to clinical trials, First edition. By A. Hackshaw. Published 2009 by Blackwell Publishing, ISBN: 978-1-4051-6774-1.

specify the ethical principles associated with conducting medical research studies of human subjects. Significant principles include:
- Informed consent must be given
- There should be prior research from animal studies
- The risks of participating in a trial should be justified by the possible benefits
- Research should be conducted by qualified health professionals
- Physical and mental harm should be avoided.

Although the Declaration is not legally binding in international law, all clinical trial protocols should state that the study has followed it. The principles have influenced legislation and regulations worldwide. For example, both the Nuremberg Code and the Declaration of Helsinki are the basis for the Code of Federal Regulations (Title 45, Volume 46),[3] issued by the US Department of Health and Human Services (DHHS) which governs federally-funded research in the US.

11.2 International Conference on Harmonisation (ICH)

The ICH guidelines[4] were developed in 1996 to harmonise the requirements for registering medicines in Europe, Japan and the United States. They are internationally recognised. As well as ensuring the safety of subjects, it allows clinical trial evidence from one country to be accepted by another, reducing many duplicate evaluations of the same treatment. The general principles of ICH expand on the Declaration of Helsinki, providing more details on the design, conduct and statistical analyses of clinical trials. ICH is divided into four major categories:

Q. Quality: Provides details on the chemical and pharmaceutical quality of the drug, such as stability, validation and impurity testing, and guidelines for Good Manufacturing Practice.

S. Safety: Provides details of the safety of the medicinal product, including toxicology and reproductive toxicology, and carcinogenicity and genotoxicity testing. It relates to *in vitro* and *in vivo* preclinical studies.

E. Efficacy: The largest section and one that is applicable to most clinical trials. It provides details of 13 core principles of Good Clinical Practice covering trial design, conduct, analysis and adverse event reporting (Box 11.1).

M. Multi-disciplinary: This section covers issues that do not fit into the other three categories, including standardised medical coding for adverse event reporting, and timing for pre-clinical studies in relation to clinical development intended to support drug registration.

11.3 Good Clinical Practice (GCP) and the EU Clinical Trials Directives

Good Clinical Practice (GCP) is a detailed set of recommendations intended to standardise clinical trial conduct. It defines the roles and responsibilities

---

Box 11.1 13 Core principles of ICH GCP guidelines for clinical trials[5]

1. Clinical trials should be conducted in accordance with the ethical principles of the Declaration of Helsinki, and consistent with Good Clinical Practice and the appropriate regulatory requirement(s).

2. A trial should only be conducted if the potential risks and inconveniences are outweighed by the expected benefit for the trial subject and society.

3. The rights, safety and well-being of trial subjects are the most important considerations and should prevail over the interests of science and society.

4. Non-clinical and clinical information about a new intervention (especially an investigational medicinal product) should be used to justify the proposed trial.

5. A clinical trial should be scientifically sound, and described in a clear and sufficiently detailed protocol.

6. A proposed trial and its protocol must have approval from an independent ethics committee. Researchers should follow the protocol when conducting the trial.

7. Trial subjects should be the responsibility of a qualified clinician (or dentist), who will make decisions about the medical care.

8. All researchers involved in conducting a trial should be qualified by education, training and experience relevant to their tasks.

9. All human subjects should give informed consent before they participate in a trial.

10. Clinical trial information should be recorded, handled and stored in a way that allows its accurate reporting, interpretation and verification.

11. Data should be kept confidential and protected, particularly when it identifies a particular subject. The regulations that govern privacy and confidentiality should be followed, where required.

12. Investigational medicinal products should be manufactured, handled and stored in accordance with Good Manufacturing Practice and used as specified in the trial protocol.

13. Systems for assuring the quality of the trial conduct and data should be in place.

---

of trial staff, while affording an appropriate level of protection to subjects. ICH[6] provides the international GCP standard, although other organisations have developed their own similar guidelines. The extent to which ICH GCP is implemented in different countries and by different researchers has been variable. This led the European Union to develop the EU Clinical Trials Directive (2001/20/EC) and associated GCP Directive (2005/28/EC) – a legal framework for clinical trial research among its member states. Some of the following sections refer to the Directives because they are detailed, cover many countries and are legally binding. However, the EU Directives, ICH GCP, and other regulations and guidelines in non-EU countries, such as those from the US FDA,[7] have much in common, so this section is applicable to researchers in all countries.

The Directives help standardise trial conduct across the EU and the European Economic Area (including Norway, Iceland and Liechtenstein), and are part of European law. They cover all clinical trials involving one or more investigational medicinal products (IMPs), and phases I to IV, but not observational studies, or interventional trials investigating a medical device, surgical technique or change in behaviour or lifestyle, though elements may be of use as examples of good practice.[#] Although there are established definitions of a clinical trial (see page 2), the EU Directives use the following terminology:[8]

A clinical trial is an investigation in human subjects which is intended to discover or verify the clinical, pharmacological and/or other pharmacodynamic effects of one or more medicinal products, identify any adverse reactions or study the absorption, distribution, metabolism and excretion, with the object of ascertaining the safety and/or efficacy of those products. This definition includes pharmacokinetic studies.

Each EU country implemented the Directives into its own legislative system. This is in addition to other laws that may already be in place, such as those associated with clinical trials of medical devices, using human tissue for research and data protection. One of the key consequences is that all trials must have a named sponsor (see Box 10.2, page 160). There are 24 'Articles', and EU Member States and sponsors have a legal obligation to meet them.[9] They cover five broad categories (Box 11.2). Some are presented in Chapter 10.

Box 11.2 Obligations covered by the EU Clinical Trials Directives

• Protect the safety and well-being of clinical trial subjects, with special reference to children and vulnerable adults

• Provide procedures to give regulatory approval before a trial starts recruiting

• Provide procedures for an independent ethics committee to review and 'approve' the trial protocol and any documentation meant for trial subjects before a trial starts recruiting and during recruitment

• Provide procedures for reporting and processing adverse events

• Specify standards for the manufacture, importing and labelling of IMPs.

[#]Individual countries may have other regulations that cover medical devices, surgical trials and trials involving exposures such as radiotherapy.

Protection of clinical trial subjects

All subjects should be protected against harm caused by being in the trial (Box 11.3). Eligible subjects must be given enough information allowing them to decide freely whether they wish to participate. This is done verbally with a health professional involved the trial, and written information (the **patient information sheet**, see page 161). If the subject decides to proceed, he/she and the health professional must sign a consent form.

Box 11.3 GCP requirements for protecting clinical trial subjects

- The expected benefits to patients or society outweigh the possible risk of harm
- The physical and mental well-being of the subject is safeguarded
- Informed consent is obtained from every trial subject or legal representative
- Subjects can withdraw from the trial at any time
- Medical care is the responsibility of a clinically qualified person (doctor or dentist)
- Subjects have a point of contact for further information about the trial at any time
- Insurance or indemnity provision must be in place to cover the liability of the investigator and sponsor.

The Directives make special reference to children (usually aged under 16 years), those who are chronically ill, the elderly, prisoners and vulnerable adults, such as those who are incapacitated, for example, mentally disabled or unconscious. This is of particular relevance where a subject is unable to give informed consent, so consent must be sought from a **legal representative**, i.e. someone who has a personal relationship with the subject, but not involved in the trial. For children, this is one or both of the parents or other legally appointed guardian, and in incapacitated adults this could be the spouse or next-of-kin.

The legal representative must be given information about the trial before providing consent. In addition, a child's view must be sought where possible, using a specially developed patient information sheet appropriate for his/her level of understanding (such as lots of simple pictures), or discussion with the health professional and parent. Incapacitated adults who later become mentally competent are able to withdraw. Whatever the method of consent used in these unusual circumstances, an ethics committee with appropriate expertise must have approved the protocol and method of recruitment.

When trials are based on children or incapacitated adults there must be a clear need for the research, the number of subjects should be as small as possible to address the main objective reliably, and efforts are needed to minimise pain, discomfort, fear and other harm.

Subjects can withdraw from the trial at any time, by discontinuing the trial treatment, or not attending clinic visits or undergoing any other assessment. Researchers can generally still use data on that subject up to the point when they withdrew, although it might be useful to make this clear in the patient information sheet and consent form. However, subjects have the right to withdraw any data that concerns them, including tissue samples, if they wish.

Insurance and indemnity

Trial sponsors normally provide insurance for **non-negligent harm** (physical or emotional injury or death) caused by participating in the trial, but where the protocol was followed correctly by site staff. This allows affected subjects to receive financial compensation from the sponsor's insurers (the sponsor would indemnify the recruiting site against such claims, i.e. the site would be protected). The patient information sheet should contain a statement about the sponsor's insurance and who to contact in the event of a claim. This insurance is different from that in a hospital, which has responsibility for the standard of care for a trial subject (where relevant). If hospital staff have been negligent, for example, they gave the wrong trial drug or dose, compensation should be met by the insurers of their employer (for **negligent harm**), and not the trial sponsor (the site would indemnify the sponsor against such claims, i.e. the sponsor would be protected). Defective drugs or medical devices should be the responsibility of the manufacturer. Details of liability and indemnity should be provided in the clinical trials agreement (see page 172). To make a negligence claim, four factors need to be established:

- A duty was owed: a legal duty exists whenever a hospital or healthcare provider undertakes care or treatment of a subject
- A duty was breached: the provider failed to conform to the relevant standard of care
- The breach caused an injury
- Damage: there needs to be a financial or emotional loss, otherwise there is no basis for a claim, even if there was negligence.

Furthermore, there may be instances where the sponsor (particularly members of the review committee who assessed the clinical trial, for example, an Institutional Review Board) or the Independent Data Monitoring Committee may be named as defendants in negligence cases, so these individuals may also need to be indemnified.

Data protection

A central database will store data about participating subjects. This often means that data will be sent out of the hospital, or other health facility, to the trial co-ordinating centre. Trial data associated with subjects such as paper case report forms (CRFs) and the electronic database should be held in a secure environment.

When people agree to participate in a trial it is on the understanding that their personal data will remain confidential, as stated in the Patient Information Sheet. Only trial staff, or other authorised parties, such as the regulatory authority, should have access to it. Also, it should not normally be necessary to easily link a subject's trial data with their name or contact details.

Many countries have regulations in place governing data protection, confidentiality, and access to personal data, for example, the EU Data Protection Directive (95/46/EC). Many trials just use a unique number to identify individuals. However, some data may not be matched to the correct patient if one digit is written down incorrectly on a CRF. A more reliable method is to add patient initials, in addition to the unique trial number.

Sometimes it is necessary to use subject names, with or without contact details. For example, in a disease prevention trial, quality of life forms may need to be posted to subjects at home because they would not normally be attending a clinic regularly. Also, where death or cancer incidence is the main trial outcome, national registries can provide a valuable source of ascertaining these events, as well as the recruiting centre, especially during long-term follow up. Clinical trial subjects are 'flagged' with the registry, so whenever they die or have been diagnosed with cancer, the trial co-ordination centre will be informed automatically. This system is often reliant on using patient names and date of birth to accurately match an event with a particular trial subject.

In any trial, collecting personal data should be justified and approved by the ethics committee, and the subject should give specific consent.

Information for subjects in foreign languages

Any documentation intended for trial subjects (e.g. patient information sheet and consent form) should be written in the dominant language(s) of the country in which subjects will be recruited. For international trials, the sponsor and lead investigator in each country should ensure that the appropriate language is used. Documentation developed by English-speaking researchers should be translated into another language, and the accuracy of this could be tested by back-translating to English to compare with the original version. The same principle applies to any language. However, it may not be worth translating the documents if few foreign-language subjects are expected. Those who are unable to sufficiently interpret the trial information may be ineligible, and this would be specified in the eligibility criteria. Alternatively, the ethics committee and institutional review board may allow a hospital translator or multilingual relative to verbally give the trial information to the subject, which could be taped so that the subjects have a record.

Regulatory approval and notification

Each country has its own regulatory authority (see Table 11.1) responsible for allowing a clinical trial to be conducted, usually studies with an IMP (or IND). The main documents to be supplied by the sponsor are listed in Box 10.6 (page 168). The application requirements differ between countries, and should be checked with the relevant authority. It is essential to obtain documented evidence of approval before subjects are recruited. Failure to do so can have legal repercussions.

Table 11.1 Regulatory agencies in selected countries.

Country	Regulatory Agency	Website
European Union*	**Competent authority in each country**	
Austria	Bundesamt für Sicherheit im Gesundheitswesen	www.ages.at
Belgium	Directoraat generaal Geneesmiddelen Direction générale Médicaments	www.afigp.fgov.be
Denmark	Lægemiddelstyrelsen	www.dkma.dk
Finland	Lääkelaitos	www.nam.fi
France	Agence Française de Sécurité Sanitaire des Produits de Santé	www.afssaps.sante.fr
Germany	Bundesministerium für Gesundheit und Soziale Sicherung Bundesinstitut für Arzneimittel und Medizinprodukte Paul-Ehrlich-Institut	www.bmgs.bund.de www.bfarm.de/de/index.php www.pei.de
Greece	National Organisation for Medicines	www.eof.gr
Iceland	Lyfjastofnun	www.lyfjastofnun.is
Ireland	Irish Medicines Board	www.imb.ie
Italy	Ministero della Salute	www.ministerosalute.it
Netherlands	Staatstoezicht op de volksgezondheid Inspectie voor de Gezondheidszorg	www.igz.nl
Norway	Statens Legemiddelverk	www.legemiddelverket.no
Portugal	Instituto Nacional da Farmácia e do Medicamento	www.infarmed.pt
Spain	Agencia española del medicamento	www.agemed.es
Sweden	Läkemedelsverket	www.lakemedelsverket.se
United Kingdom	Medicines and Healthcare products Regulatory Agency	www.mhra.gov.uk
Czech Republic	State Institute for Drug Control Institute for the State Control of Veterinary Biologicals and Medicaments	www.uskvbl.cz www.sukl.cz
Hungary	National Institute of Pharmacy Institute for Veterinary Medicinal Products	www.ogyi.hu
Poland	Office for Medicinal Products	www.urpl.gov.pl
Australia	Therapeutic Goods Administration	www.tga.gov.au
Canada	Health Canada	www.hc-sc.gc.ca/
China	State Food and Drug Administration	eng.sfda.gov.cn/eng/
India	Drugs Controller General of India, the Central Drugs Standard Control Organization	cdsco.nic.in/
Japan	Pharmaceutical and Medical Devices Agency	www.pmda.go.jp/index-e.html www.mhlw.go/jp/english/index.html
United States	Food and Drug Administration	www.fda.gov

For further details on trial set up in European countries, use the following website (replace 'France' with another European country)

http://www.efgcp.be/Downloads/EFGCPReportFiles/Flow%20chart%20France%20 (revised)%2007-09-01.pdf

Summaries of regulations that govern clinical trials, regulatory bodies and ethics review processes in EU countries are found on the European Forum GCP website (given below Table 11.1). During the trial, the regulatory authority or IRB usually needs to be notified of any major change to the trial design or conduct.

Independent ethics committee assessment

Proposed trials need be reviewed by an independent ethics committee, comprising of a group of experts who are able to assess the trial, including the protocol and all material intended for subjects (see page 169). Recruitment should not begin until written confirmation of ethics approval is received. Sometimes it is necessary for the ethics committee to seek additional expertise when, for example, trials are based on children, or incapacitated or other vulnerable adults. This is a requirement of the EU Clinical Trials Directives. In the US, ethics can be assessed by an Institutional Review Board (IRB), which also reviews the scientific merit of the proposed study, protocol and other documentation such as the Investigator's Brochure.

Procedures for reporting and processing adverse events

There should be a system for identifying and reporting adverse events (see page 181). The regulations in most countries are associated with IMP trials, but they may also apply to other interventions, such as medical devices. Many countries have similar procedures for classifying adverse events according to severity, whether unexpected or not and the timelines for reporting them to the regulatory authority. It is good practice to collect information on safety for any trial. Even if no adverse events were observed, the final report is strengthened by stating that an attempt was made to collect this data.

In the EU there is now a **Eudra Vigilance Database**[10] containing safety information about all IMPs used in EU clinical trials, and based on SUSAR reporting and annual safety reports. The database allows this information to be exchanged more easily between countries that use it.

Specify standards for the manufacturing, importing and labelling of IMPs (INDs)

Sponsors of IMP clinical trials must ensure that the trial drugs are manufactured to a high standard, and stored and labelled correctly (see page 170), in accordance with the internationally recognised guidelines for Good Manufacturing Practice (GMP), a set of standards for the management of manufacturing and quality control of medicinal products.[11]

In the EU, there is a legal requirement for IMP trials to be conducted in accordance with GMP (GMP Directive 91/356/EEC). Licensed products are released in accordance with their marketing authorisation. For unlicensed products, or licensed drugs that are manipulated in any way (including their packaging), at least one qualified person (QP) should have responsibility for releasing them to hospitals or subjects, and for maintaining records. For drugs manufactured in or imported into the EU, only one QP is required to 'sign off' distribution throughout Europe.

11.4 Independent audit or inspection of clinical trials

Many countries have a system for inspecting clinical trials facilities, i.e. the offices and working practices of the sponsor, the trial co-ordinating centre, one or more of the recruiting sites, and drug manufacturing facilities. This is a legal requirement of the EU Clinical Trials Directives, and can be made before, during or after a trial is conducted, arising from a pre-planned inspection or triggered because of an unexpected and urgent serious concern. A single trial or several trials can be inspected during a visit.

An inspection team attend in person. They assess compliance with the national regulations, ensuring that:
- The necessary regulatory and ethical approvals, and signed agreements were obtained
- The trial documentation (e.g. Trial Master File, see page 175) is available, complete and up-to-date
- GCP guidelines are followed adequately
- Systems are in place for monitoring compliance with the trial protocol
- There are clear systems for monitoring safety, and serious adverse events are reported on time.

The inspectors interview relevant staff and produce a report detailing any problems found. If there are serious issues with the trial, especially if they significantly affect the safety of subjects, inspectors have the authority to suspend the trial.

11.5 Regulations surrounding research in special populations

The EU, US and several other countries have regulations for research in special populations. For example, there 5,000 to 8,000 distinct rare diseases that affect 6–8% of the US population. They are known as orphan diseases and, until recently, people suffering from such diseases had little recourse available to them. This was because pharmaceutical companies did not find it profitable to spend the money needed to research and develop drugs in these areas. The governments of some countries now provide incentives to companies to encourage the development of these drugs. For example, the regulatory authority would grant a company a period of market exclusivity (7 years in the US, or 10 years in the EU), during which time, the company is assured of sale of the drug without competition, provided certain caveats are met. Companies now have the incentive to invest money in researching rare diseases, and this includes many biotechnology companies.

The EU and FDA also have laws and regulations surrounding the research and development of drugs for use in children (generally aged 0 to 17). Regulation EC No. 1901/2006 or the 'Pediatric Regulation' is designed to better protect the health of children in EU trials.

11.6 Non-EU countries

Many aspects of the regulations and guidelines are similar between countries.

United States

Two principle sets of regulations that govern clinical trials in the US come from the FDA and the Department of Health and Human Services. The FDA regulations are the most commonly used. It is the national regulatory agency in the US, providing extensive documentation for researchers on its website.

A trial drug is called an Investigational New Drug (IND). A sponsor must file an application with the FDA at least 30 days before initiating a trial that evaluates a new drug for the first time in humans. It contains quality and safety data about the drug from animal and laboratory studies to give assurance that it can be used safely when administered in accordance with the trial protocol. An IND is considered approved unless the FDA objects within the 30-day period. The sponsor must submit annual reports on the status of the trial. Subsequent studies can be conducted with the same IND, provided the sponsor submits all the required paperwork to the FDA.

There are several laws, including the Food, Drug and Cosmetic Act and those listed in Chapter 21 of the Code of Federal Regulations.[12] Procedures for trial set-up and conduct follow ICH GCP closely, and therefore have been largely covered above. Trials are reviewed by an Institutional Review Board (IRB) from each centre where subjects will be recruited. Board members cannot be part of the research team. Some central IRBs cover several sites. The IRB reviews the protocol, investigator's brochure and documentation for subjects, and the ethical considerations.

Sponsors should be responsible for quality assurance of the IND, including quality control and distribution. Safety reporting is similar to European trials, in which serious adverse event reports and IND Annual Reports are sent to the FDA, and the timelines are similar to those in Europe (see page 181). Major changes to the protocol or to the other information submitted for the IND, and addition of new investigators participating in the study must also be reported to the FDA by filing timely amendments.

Inspections are part of the Bioresearch Monitoring Program. Although the FDA cannot enforce its regulations outside of the US, it can and does penalise sponsors who wish to obtain FDA approval of a marketing application if they have used non-compliant clinical sites outside the US.

In order to identify and minimise investigator bias associated with the trial, sponsors submitting a marketing application for a medicinal product must provide information on compensation to, and financial interests of, all the investigators who participated in the clinical trial used in the application. This requires applicants to confirm that the investigators have no financial interests in the drug or the sponsoring company, or to disclose any financial arrangements. If the sponsor does not provide this information, the FDA can refuse to file the application.

Under FDA legislation (FDA Amendments Act of 2007) clinical trial results must be posted on www.clinicaltrials.gov. Previously the information on the study design and recruitment were posted on the website, but in the interest of public disclosure of both positive and negative data, the FDA now requires the results to be publicly available.

Canada

Trials that involve a pharmaceutical, biological, or radiopharmaceutical drug must obtain approval via a Clinical Trials Application, from Health Canada, the regulatory authority. The law that governs the use of clinical trial drugs is the Controlled Drugs and Substances Act. The system for trial set-up and conduct is similar to the United States and Europe.

The Health Products and Food Branch Inspectorate (HPFBI) aims to inspect all institutions that conduct clinical trials. Further details about trial set-up and conduct in Canada can be obtained from their regulatory website.[13]

Japan

The medicinal products market in Japan is among the largest in the world, and there is a long history of clinical trial research. There was once a view that Japanese subjects reacted to drugs in a different way from other nationalities, so there was a tendency to repeat trials conducted elsewhere. However, with ICH GCP, there is now a high degree of standardisation with the US and EU, and the original guidelines for trial set-up and conduct have been considerably revised.

The national regulatory agency is the Pharmaceutical and Medical Devices Agency (PMDA), and a key regulation is the Pharmaceutical Affairs Law (1996). ICH GCP compliance is a legal requirement. Researchers (or their sponsor) must submit a Clinical Trial Plan Notification to the PMDA before recruitment begins. Sponsors are encouraged to have an in-house study review board to evaluate the proposed trial. However, the trial must be approved, and reviewed annually by an IRB for each recruiting site. Sometimes, several sites share an IRB. During the trial, suspected unexpected serious adverse reactions (SUSARs) must be reported to the Ministry of Health, Labour and Welfare (MHLW), in a similar way to European trials (see page 181). Audits and inspections are the responsibility of the sponsor. Further details are found on the websites in Table 11.1 and reference 14.

Australia

Australia was considered when the ICH GCP guidelines were first developed, so elements of trial set-up and conduct are similar. The regulatory body is the Therapeutic Goods Administration (TGA). The laws that govern clinical trials include the Therapeutic Goods Act (1989), the Therapeutic Goods Regulations (1990) and the Therapeutic Goods (Medical Devices) Regulations (2002). IMPs or investigational medical devices, are both referred to as 'unapproved therapeutic goods', and include new and unlicensed drugs, or those that are already licensed (and appear on the Australian Register of Therapeutic Goods) but will be used in a 'separate and distinct' way.

Unlicensed treatments must be granted a Clinical Trial Notification (CTN) or Clinical Trial Exemption (CTX) before they can be used in a trial. All trials require ethics approval by one of the human research ethics committees (HRECs), and the Australian Health Ethics Committee of the National Health and Medical Research Council must be informed of trials of unapproved therapeutic goods. In drug or medical device manufacturing, import, labelling and testing, the sponsor must provide certificates of analysis and ensure compliance with Good Manufacturing Practice.

The reporting of serious adverse events to the regulatory body (TGA) is practically the same as in Europe (see page 181), including annual safety reports. The TGA can also inspect any organisation involved in trial conduct. Further details can be obtained from websites.[15,16]

China

With over 1.3 billion people, China is a potentially large source of trial subjects and there are several 'mega trials' being conducted, based on many thousands of people. The cost of conducting trials is relatively low, and with the ability to recruit large numbers of patients quite quickly, the number of trials is increasing, particularly through international collaboration. However, clinical trial research is still relatively new in China and local staff need to become familiar with conducting trials to international standards. China has its own guidelines for GCP, based on ICH GCP. Clinical trials of IMPs and medical devices are regulated by the State Food and Drug Administration (SFDA), and they need to comply with the Drug Administration Law (2001) and the Drug Registration Procedure (2002).

The process for trial set-up has been streamlined, and there are clear rules for assuring the rights and interests of subjects, such as obtaining signed consent (directly or from an authorised representative). Only sites that have GCP certification are allowed to participate in trials. Clinical trial applications are submitted to the SFDA, which reviews aspects such as inspection of sites, assessment of the trial drugs or medical devices, and ethics approval. The Centre for Drug Evaluation (CDE) makes a technical evaluation of the drugs. The entire process may take at least three months, but trials cannot start until approval is received from the SFDA. Reporting of serious adverse events is similar to elsewhere (see website in Table 11.1).

India

India, like China, has a large population and can conduct trials relatively cheaply. The regulatory body is the Drugs Controller General of India (DCGI) and trials of IMPs and medical devices are governed by the Drugs and Cosmetics Act (revised Schedule Y 2003). Researchers are expected largely to comply with guidelines for trial set-up and conduct from the US FDA. The DCGI can grant permission to conduct a trial without prior ethics committee approval, but researchers are requested not to recruit subjects until this is obtained. During the trial, serious adverse reactions need to be reported to the DCGI and the ethics committee within 14 days of discovery. Continual approval is conditional on yearly reports. When reviewing the submitted protocol, the DCGI may seek advice from the Indian Council of Medical Research.[17] During the trial, any changes to the protocol must be reported to the DCGI and permission sought for major changes. The Indian regulatory agency is preparing to streamline the clinical research process and, with the help of US FDA, is planning to set up a Central Drug Authority in the near future. Further details can be obtained from one of the national websites,[18] and the website in Table 11.1.

11.7 Summary

There are key regulatory issues associated with trial set-up and conduct:
• Informed consent
• Good Clinical Practice
• Good Manufacturing Practice
• National regulatory approval (review trial protocol and investigator's brochure)
• Institutional and/or ethics committee approval
• Monitoring and reporting adverse events (serious adverse events that are judged to be caused by the trial treatment are reported to the regulatory authority)
• Provision for compensation to trial subjects if they suffer harm because of being in the trial.

References

1. http://ohsr.od.nih.gov/guidelines/nuremberg.html
2. http://www.wma.net/e/policy/b3.htm
3. http://www.access.gpo.gov/nara/cfr/waisidx_00/45cfr46_00.html
4. http://www.ich.org/cache/compo/276-254-1.html
5. http://www.ich.org/LOB/media/MEDIA482.pdf (see page 8).
6. www.ich.org
7. http://www.fda.gov/oc/gcp/default.htm
8. http://www.mhra.gov.uk/Howweregulate/Medicines/Licensingof-medicines/Clinicaltrials/Isaclinicaltrialauthorisationrequired/index.htm

9. http://ec.europa.eu/enterprise/pharmaceuticals/eudralex/vol-1/dir_2001_20/dir_2001_20_en.pdf#

10. http://eudravigilance.emea.europa.eu/veterinary/evDbms01.asp

11. http://www.ich.org/LOB/media/MEDIA433.pdf

12. http://www.access.gpo.gov/nara/cfr/cfr-table-search.html#page1

13. http://www.hc-sc.gc.ca/dhp-mps/prodpharma/applic-demande/guide-ld/clini/index_e.html

14. Griffin JP, O'Grady J (Eds). *The Textbook of Pharmaceutical Medicine*. 5th edn. BMJ Books, Blackwell Publishing, 2006.

15. http://www.qctn.com.au/ConductingTrials/HowtostartatrialinAustralia/tabid/67/Default.aspx

16. http://www.qctn.com.au/Portals/0/Australian%20Clinical%20Trials-%20Handbook.pdf

17. http://www.icmr.nic.in/

18. http://www.iscr.org/ClinicalTrialsRegulation.aspx

Reading list

Altman D. *Practical Statistics for Medical Research*. CRC Press, 1990.

Altman D, Machin D, Bryant TN, Gardner MJ. *Statistics With Confidence*. 2nd edn. BMJ Books, 2000.

Bland JM. *An Introduction to Medical Statistics*. 3rd edn. Oxford University Press, 2000.

Clive C. *Handbook of SOPs for Good Clinical Practice*. 2nd edn. Interpharm Press Inc., 2004.

Ellenbery S, Fleming TR, DeMets DL. *Data Monitoring Committees in Clinical Trials: A Practical Perspective (Statistics in Practice)*. John Wiley & Sons, Ltd, 2002.

Friedman L, Furberg CD, DeMets DL. *Fundamentals of Clinical Trials*. 3rd Rev. edn. Springer-Verlag New York Inc., 2006.

Girling D, Parmar M, Stenning S, Stephens R, Stewart, L. *Clinical Trials in Cancer: Principles and Practice*. Oxford University Press, 2003.

Griffin JP, O'Grady J (Eds). *The Textbook of Pharmaceutical Medicine*. 5th edn. BMJ Books, Blackwell Publishing, 2006.

Guyatt G, Rennie D, Meade M, Cook D. *Users' Guides to the Medical Literature: A Manual for Evidence-Based Clinical Practice*. 2nd edn. McGraw-Hill Medical, 2008.

Kirkwood B, Sterne J. *Medical Statistics*. 2nd edn. Blackwell, 2003.

Machin D, Day S, Green S, Everitt B, George S (Eds). *Textbook of Clinical Trials*. John Wiley & Sons, Ltd, 2004.

Petrie A, Sabin C. *Medical Statistics at a Glance*. 2nd edn. BMJ Books, 2005.

Pocock S. *Clinical Trials: A Practical Approach*. John Wiley & Sons, Ltd, 1983.

Sackett DL, Straus SE, Richardson WS, Rosenberg W, Haynes RB. *Evidence-Based Medicine: How to Practice and Teach EBM*. 2nd Rev. edn. Churchill Livingstone, 2000.

Statistical formulae for calculating some 95% confidence intervals

95% confidence interval = effect size $\pm$ 1.96 × standard error of the effect size

Single-arm phase II trial
Counting people (single proportion)

Number of responses to treatment = 28

Number of subjects (N) = 50

Observed proportion (P) = 28/50 = 0.56 (or 56%)

Standard error of the true proportion (SE) = $\sqrt{[P \times (1 - P)]/N} =$

$\sqrt{(0.56 \times 0.44)/50} = 0.07$

95% CI = P $\pm$ 1.96 × SE = 0.56 $\pm$ 1.96 × 0.07 = 0.42 to 0.70 (or 42 to 70%)

For small trials (e.g. $N < 30$) 'exact' methods provide a more accurate 95% confidence interval (Geigy Scientific Tables. *Introduction to Statistics, Statistics Tables and Mathematical Formulae*, 8th edn. Ciba Geigy, 1982).

Taking measurements on people (single mean value)

Mean value ($\bar{x}$) = 34 mm (VAS score)

Standard deviation (s) = 18 mm

Number of subjects (N) = 40

Standard error (SE) = $\dfrac{s}{\sqrt{n}} = 18/\sqrt{40} = 2.8$ mm

95% CI = mean $\pm$ 1.96 × SE = 34 $\pm$ 1.96 × 2.8 = 34 $\pm$ 5.5 = 28 to 40 mm

For small trials ($N < 30$), a different multiplier to 1.96 is used. It comes from the 't-distribution', and gets larger as the sample size gets smaller

The multiplier of 1.96 is associated with a two-sided confidence interval. For a one-sided limit a value of 1.645 could be used, but only the lower or upper limit is needed, depending on whether the proportion or mean associated with the new therapy should be greater or smaller than standard treatments to indicate improvement.

Randomised phase II or III trial with two groups

Counting people (risk difference or relative risk)
Example is serological flu (Box 7.1)

$P_1 = r_1/N_1 = 41/927 = 0.044$

$P_2 = r_2/N_2 = 80/911 = 0.088$

For risk difference

Observed risk difference $= P_1 - P_2 = -0.044 \, (-4.4\%)$

Standard error (SE) $= \sqrt{\{[P_1 \times (1 - P_1)]/N_1 + [P_2 \times (1 - P_2)]/N_2\}} = 0.01155$

95% CI $=$ difference $\pm 1.96 \times$ SE $= -0.044 \pm 1.96 \times 0.01155$

$= -0.066$ to $-0.021 = -6.6\%$ to -2.1%

For relative risk (RR)

Observed RR $= P_1 \div P_2 = 0.5$

Take natural logarithm (base e) $= \log_e (0.5) = -0.693$

Standard error of the log RR (SE) $= \sqrt{(1/r_1 + 1/r_2 - 1/N_1 - 1/N_2)} = 0.186$

95% CI for the log RR $=$ log RR $\pm 1.96 \times$ SE

$= -0.693 \pm 1.96 \times 0.186 = -1.058$ to -0.328

Transform back (take exponential) $= 0.35$ to 0.72 (i.e. $e^{-1.058}$ to $e^{-0.328}$)

('e' is the natural number 2.71828)

Converted to a percentage change in risk, 95% CI is 28 to 65% reduction in risk

Taking measurements on people (difference between two mean values)
Example is the Atkins diet (Box 7.4)

Change in weight loss at three months

Atkins diet:	$N_1 = 33$	Mean$_1 = -6.8$ kg	$SD_1 = 5.0$ kg
Conventional diet:	$N_2 = 30$	Mean$_2 = -2.7$ kg	$SD_2 = 3.7$ kg

Difference between the two means $=$ Mean$_1 -$ Mean$_2 = -6.8 - (-2.7) = -4.1$ kg

Standard error of the mean difference (SE) $= \sqrt{(SD_1^2/N_1 + SD_2^2/N_2)}$

$= \sqrt{(5.0^2/33 + 3.7^2/30)} = 1.1$

95% CI $=$ mean difference $\pm 1.96 \times$ SE

$= -4.1 \pm 1.96 \times 1.1 = -6.3$ to -1.9 kg

1.96 is used when each trial group has at least say 30 subjects. For smaller studies, a larger multiplier and the t-distribution are used, and there is a different formulae depending on whether the standard deviations are similar between the groups.

Time-to-event data (hazard ratio)

A statistical package should be used to estimate 95% CIs because the calculation for the standard error is not simple. However, if only the median and number of events in each treatment group are available, there is a simple method to obtain an approximate estimate of the CI, but only after assuming that the distribution of the time-to-event measure has an 'exponential distribution' (i.e. the event rate is constant over time).

Example is early vs late radiotherapy in treating lung cancer (Spiro *et al.*, *J Clin Oncol* 2006; **24**: 3823–3830), and the outcome is time to death:

Early radiotherapy:

Median survival M1 = 13.7 months   Number of deaths = E1 = 135

Late radiotherapy:

Median survival M2 = 15.1 months   Number of deaths = E2 = 136

Hazard ratio (early vs late) HR = M2/M1 = 15.1/13.7 = 1.10

Standard error of the log hazard ratio (SE) = $\sqrt{(1/\,E1 + 1/\,E2)}$

$\quad = \sqrt{(1/135 + 1/136)} = 0.1215$

95% CI for the log HR = loge HR $\pm$ 1.96 $\times$ SE

$\quad = \log(1.10) \pm 1.96 \times 0.1215 = -0.143$ to 0.333

Transform back (take exponential) $= 0.87$ to 1.40 (i.e. $e^{-0.143}$ to $e^{0.333}$)

These are close, but not identical, to the results calculated using the raw data: HR = 1.16, 95% CI 0.91 to 1.47

Index

EU: European Union.